Delay and Pray ™

Delay and Pray™

PERMANENT WEIGHT LOSS
THROUGH SPIRITUAL FASTING

BETH BUBIK

bel esprit books
Dallas | Fort Worth

Delay and Pray™: Permanent Weight Loss Through Spiritual Fasting
Beth Bubik

Copyright © 2024 Beth Bubik

Published by Bel Esprit Books, LLC
PO Box 821801
North Richland Hills, TX 76182

The views and positions expressed in this book are those of the author and do not necessarily reflect the views and positions of the publisher.

Scripture taken from the SAINT JOSEPH NEW CATHOLIC BIBLE® Copyright © 2019 by Catholic Book Publishing Corp. Used with permission. All rights reserved.

Cover and interior design and typesetting: Kent Jensen | knail.com
Illustrations: Mary Catherine Walter
Cover photos: Shutterstock
Author photo: Mike Mitchell

ISBN: 9798218396619

First Edition: April 2024

CONTENTS

WHAT OTHERS ARE SAYING ABOUT *DELAY AND PRAY™*

Fasting was a central practice of Catholic life—alongside prayer and the sacraments—for fifteen hundred years. But in the last few centuries, it's almost entirely disappeared, but for a few symbolic remnants on Ash Wednesday, Good Friday, and an hour before Mass!

Is it any wonder the Church, and our culture, are in such peril? And is it merely a coincidence that our culture is now awash in "diseases of civilization"—such as diabetes and obesity?

Unfortunately, most Catholics can't imagine real fasting, and assume it must be torture. In truth, it's a skill—a discipline—that can be learned. It should be a sacrifice. It's not meant to be torture. And done right, it can transform both your spiritual and bodily health.

But all new disciplines require small, simple acts that can become habits. That's where Beth Bubik's *Delay and Pray™* shines through. If you follow her advice in this book, fasting—and real feasting!—will soon be a permanent part of your life. And your life will be better and richer because of it.

—**JAY RICHARDS**, PhD, Author of *Eat, Fast, Feast*, Director of The Richard and Helen DeVos Center for Life, Religion, and Family, and the William E. Simon Senior Research Fellow in American Principles and Public Policy

As a Catholic mental health clinician, I have carried grave concerns regarding the positive correlation between the rise of a great need for mental health support and healing among the members of the Body of Christ and the rise of coach and mentoring ministers who at times are falling short of the discipline, expertise and training that the people of God deserve. Beth, through her *Delay and Pray*™ Catholic coaching ministry, stands out and apart as the exception. Beth has taken the lead in establishing a professional identity for Catholic coaches that deploys the unique gifts of that field with discipline and care, while respecting and running alongside the field of mental health. In her book, she demonstrates her fidelity not only to mental health excellence as it is addressed in her coaching model, but also nutritional education excellence, and above all an excellence in communicating and sharing the rich traditions of our Catholic faith available to us as we strive for wholeness and virtue. In *Delay and Pray*™, Beth is willing to get down under your cross of overeating with you and generously share the gifts she has reaped from the soil of her own life and education. She helps you move toward freedom as children of God.

—**SISTER JOSEPHINE GARRETT**,
Sister of the Holy Family of Nazareth, Licensed
Counselor, Author & Host of the Hope Stories Podcast

Delay and Pray™ is way more than a weight loss hack. It's the key to unlocking the full transformative effects of the Gospel. While Beth's simple and practical method outlined in this book can certainly help you meet your goals for greater physical health, the most pleasant surprise is in the unexpected encounter with Christ in your places of deepest longing. A must read!

—**ERIN AND MATT INGOLD**, Owners of Metanoia Catholic

Have you ever struggled with dieting or fasting for a particular faith petition, but instead of thinking of Jesus, you focus on your next meal? If you have, like me, then this book is just for you! Beth Bubik guides you through a fabulous spiritual journey that helps you transform the 'torture of fasting' into a 'testimony of faith in action', fulfilling intentions, and getting holy and healthy at the same time. Enjoy this wonderful book!

—**SR. DEIRDRE M. BYRNE**, POSC Superior of Washington, DC Convent

To the Blessed Mother
who called me to fasting for years
before I finally answered.

To my own Mother who helped
me answer that call just before she died.

To my husband, Mike, the love of my life,
and Nick, Katy, Alyssa, and Mark and their families,
the little loves that fill my heart.

To the whole world: know that there is
always something that you can do to change yourself,
your family, and the world. You can fast and pray
and miracles will happen!

DISCLAIMER

This book contains general information and advice related to the potential benefits of fasting. It presents the research and ideas of its author. It is not intended to be a substitute for consultation with a professional healthcare practitioner. Consult with your doctor or professional healthcare practitioner before beginning any diet changes or supplemental regimen. The publisher and the author disclaim responsibility for any adverse effects resulting directly or indirectly from any information that is contained in the book.

INTRODUCTION

My life has been beautifully enhanced by Spiritual Fasting. Not only enhanced, but transformed from year to year. I had always wanted to fast on bread and water for the Blessed Mother and her intentions, but could never form a consistent routine or Rule of Life around praying and fasting until I became a Catholic Life and Weight Coach. It was in this space that I learned to manage my mind, and everything finally came together.

I am an engineer by degree and a teacher by another degree so I love to solve problems in the most creative way. I enjoy being organized and making things simple to follow, repeatable, and deeply meaningful. Hence, the Delay and Pray™ method was born. In this book, I will teach it to you, giving you a foundation for Spiritual Fasting, including how to do it, and why. Delaying and praying may be a bit challenging to adopt, but when the method is understood, it is liberating and easy to adhere to forever. This is the way to invite Jesus and the Blessed Mother into your weight and health struggles.

My own mother would have *loved* this whole process. She was my inspiration for creating the Delay and Pray™ method, and she continues to be to this day. Her name is Joanne Bauer. She was a hoot! You could always find her cooking with a smile, usually sitting on her step stool in the kitchen, while peeling potatoes or dicing vegetables for soup.

My Mom was a fantastic cook and could cobble together meals on a dime and within a very short amount of time. I remember when spaghetti sauce in a jar was first advertised on television, she said, "Oh, gosh, that will never catch on! Who would spend the money on that when making spaghetti sauce from scratch is so easy?"

She always had a garden, and we'd eat a salad before meals. We were expected at the dinner table in the evenings for "supper." There was always a pot of soup or stew on the stove, and she'd often say that "she loved us through our stomachs." My Mom fasted off sweets most of her life for the sanctity of her family, and we feasted on Sundays with a tiny glass of orange juice and one piece of bacon each with pancakes and eggs after Mass. Orange juice and bacon were premium items back in the day.

This is how I grew up—savoring the little things.

We ate, we fasted, and we feasted.

When I became a wife and mother, my Mom taught me everything I know about meals in general: how to prepare well in advance, how to use leftovers to make more meals, how to portion the meals, and how she did it all for $50 a week for eight children and a husband!

Cheers to you, Mom! You are the one person in my life that I can say loved me absolutely unconditionally. How fortunate I am to have had you for my mother and friend. I miss you and will see you again in heaven one day.

And now, to celebrate my first book, it is my honor to conclude this introduction with my Mom's words from her cookbook, created in 2001.

May you grow ever closer to Jesus as you Delay and Pray™,

—Beth Bubik
Union, Michigan
January 2024

Our family meals were the most important part of our day. It was the one time where we all sat down together, prayed, and talked about what happened to each one of us. Sharing and laughing together, "breaking bread," sometimes crying also, bonded us as a family, creating warm ties of friendship and love that can't be forgotten.

Every holiday was a wonderful celebration, always around a table of food. Whenever there was a party, graduation, Communion, Baptism, weddings, it was always celebrated around the banquet table, so what goes on at church also goes on in the home. The Eucharist begins around the family tables with the simplest of prayers, helping us understand what Christian means by "breaking bread" and "sharing a cup in Jesus' name." Ultimately, we love and serve our Lord by loving, serving and helping one another.

I can't remember when I started to wear an apron, it is such a part of my attire now.

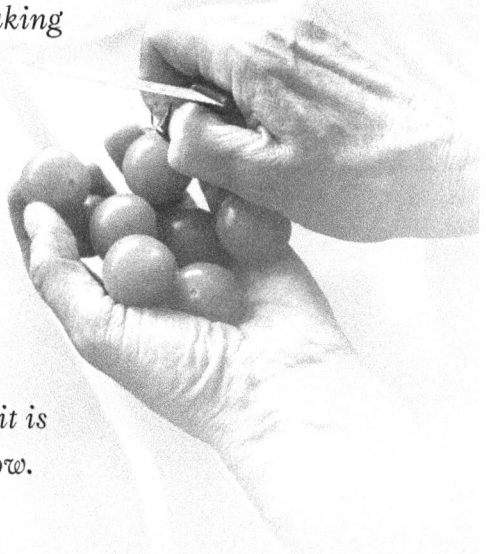

As I dress in the morning and I put on my apron, it's as if I'm saying, "I am ready to serve." Even Jim had an apron to don when he grilled! So, as we cooked our meals through the years and special recipes were handed down from generation to generation, traditions formed.

Smells of cooking brought back memories of other times. Some of our ancestors have passed on but as we look at the recipes, it's like we're visited by a "communion of saints," women whose essence fills our lives with their goodness and love and memories.

When Christmas approaches, we start to think of baking—how many can remember doing this with your Grandmother? As you begin again this coming year, I bet you'll feel their presence, and it'll give you a spiritual energy you can't imagine. As our favorite recipes are passed on, we must remember Jesus reminding us of the importance of tradition when He said "Do this in memory of me."

Looking forward to more warm memories, family traditions, I remain lovingly, Wife, Mother, Aunt, Grandma, Great Grandma, and Friend.

—Joanne Bauer

CHAPTER 1

The Promise of Delay and Pray™

"Come to me, all you who are weary and
overburdened, and I will give you rest. Take my yoke
upon you and learn from me, for I am meek and
humble of heart and you will find rest for your souls,
For my yoke is easy and my burden is light."
—Matthew 11:28-30

YOUR OLD DIET IS not working. In fact, can we have a rest from dieting altogether? Can we throw the diet mentality out the window for good? Let's just be done with it.

Traditional dieting is self-focused, too hard, and often only produces temporary results. The mentality required is chock-full of self-reliance, scarcity, and pressure to achieve a weight goal by your own white-knuckling work.

So take a breath.

This is different. You are being invited onto a new and wonderful weight loss path. This journey of health will actually get you where you want to go because you will be holding the hand of Jesus while learning to delay unhealthy foods and pray for others through it all. You will drop the weight for good and find joy in the challenge, too.

I call this unique process Delay and Pray™. You will be delaying sugar, flour, and alcohol (SFA) until Sundays through prayer and Spiritual Fasting. The Delay and Pray™ method of Spiritual Fasting is the road to reaching your dreams and taking your loved ones with you in prayer. This program works because you will be putting the souls of others before your own. It is what you were created for—to love your neighbor as yourself.[1]

Delaying and praying. That's the entire program in a nutshell.

It is simple, but it is not easy. Because there are days when delaying and praying will feel like suffering. And you have to be taught how to suffer well. Suffering well is a skill that can be intentionally practiced. Most of us are terrible at it and don't even try to improve. But you will soon discover that suffering well is redemptive for you and others because Jesus is at the center of it. He meets you in your need.

I have been following the Delay and Pray™ method for a few years now. I developed this program because I was desperate to stop overeating and overdrinking. At the same time, there were things happening in my life that I knew deep in my heart only God could fix. One day, I figured out how to put prayer and fasting together in a way that halts all the "over-ing" by putting a slow stop to emotional eating and drinking. At first I did it out of passion to help someone I loved, and then I did it for the good of my body and soul. When the miracles started happening, I realized that prayer combined with fasting changes the lives of others. That's when my life started to explode with blessings. I'm so thankful God showed me the way to Spiritual Fasting.

In this book, I'll show you the way. But before we begin, there are two promises I want to make.

My first promise is that you will feel better very soon.

Over time, you are going to lose weight permanently while growing closer to God. But you can actually choose to feel a little better right now, before any of your behaviors or results change. This is possible by inviting Jesus into your holistic health with a new body-and-soul approach, trusting that He will give you the grace for each step. His yoke is easy, and His burden is light.[2] He is the one thing that is certain.

So, trust Him.

You are not alone, and
God works where you can't.

You will also feel better because you are going to start praying for miracles ... right now. This is a journey, and even as you are learning, you will help those you love with your prayers and intentions. The very act of praying for others from Day One will cause you to succeed. Trust Jesus to start bringing miracles through your prayers immediately. You are not alone, and God works where you can't.

The second promise is that you will learn how to do hard things.

In fact, you will learn how to do the hardest thing of all: forgive yourself when you make a mistake.

Remember the biblical passage when Peter asks Jesus if he needs to forgive others as many as seven times? The Lord answered him, "I say to you, not seven times, but seventy times seven" (Matt 18:22).

> *It's time to forgive yourself
> seventy times seven.*

Jesus wasn't suggesting that we need to keep an accurate count of the faults we have forgiven. He was implying that we need to forgive endlessly. Now, that's hard! And as challenging as it is to forgive others endlessly, it is even harder to forgive ourselves endlessly. But you can learn.

It's time to forgive yourself seventy times seven.

I refer to this concept as *Nunc Coepi*. It is a Latin phrase that means "to begin again with gentle repentance." Venerable Bruno Lateri writes, "If I should fall even a thousand times a day, a thousand times, with peaceful repentance, I will say immediately, 'Nunc Coepi' [Now I begin]."[3]

This phrase is helpful because there are days when you will overeat this or overdrink that, but you can forgive yourself with gentle repentance and begin again. You can even have a good cry about it, but get right back up and Nunc Coepi. The Delay and Pray™ method is different from anything you've tried so look at yourself through the eyes of Jesus and give yourself grace. This means saying, "I'm sorry" to yourself and to Jesus then starting to do better right that moment.

Not tomorrow.

Not on Monday morning.

Now.

Gentle repentance will begin with food and alcohol consumption and then permeate through everything you do. It is the beginning of a whole new virtuous life. You will be forever changed by the process itself, not just by achieving a thinner body, wearing a new wardrobe, and receiving many answered prayers. You will be richer in soul because your transformation will happen from the inside out.

Filled with virtue by the grace of God, you will lean into discomfort, expect it, and embrace it instead of eating and drinking your way out of it. You will not only learn to feel the discomfort, but to use it as prayer to heal your family, spouse, job situation, health, parish priest, and friends. The possibilities are endless so you must forgive yourself endlessly.

As I see it, there are two options that are always in front of you. One way is to waste your current discomfort by eating and drinking your way out of it. Your brain will want to choose this very familiar path.

This second option is Spiritual Fasting, and it is the better path. Along this path, you will begin losing weight, obtaining optimal health, and letting Jesus transform your suffering while you bring your children back to Church, experience financial breakthroughs, and maybe even heal the problems of the nation. It can be done.

Jesus and Mary will be walking with you on this journey. I'm also walking with you, along with a whole community of Spiritual Fasters.

Are you ready?

To begin, let's go back to the place where Jesus shows us how to carry our suffering. Come to the dusty and jagged road of Calvary where Jesus Christ was under the tremendous weight of the cross, suffering for the salvation of the world. With great pain, He carried the wood that would eventually bear His crucifixion and death. This very wood would also be an eternal symbol of His resurrection. Jesus sanctifies everything He touches.

If you let Him into your struggles, He will sanctify those, too.

Enter Simon of Cyrene, an ordinary man of his time, who was pressed into service beside Jesus under the heavy cross of salvation. Soldiers pulled him from the crowd and thrust him onto the violent scene without consent. There are some accounts that claim Simon was no stranger to hatred, as he had just experienced the death of his family at the hands of Roman soldiers.[4]

> *Jesus sanctifies everything He touches. If you let Him into your struggles, He will sanctify those, too.*

Simon of Cyrene was like all of us. He was full of emotion and confusion as he suffered alongside our Savior in shared pain on their dangerous and rocky journey. We can surmise that he didn't really understand Jesus or what the crucifixion was all about. We know that he didn't want to be there. As he traveled with Jesus, he experienced both the Roman brutality and the compassion of Christian onlookers beside the road. Along the way, Simon's strength of body and soul was transformed to help bear the heavy cross.

I can only imagine Simon's arm around the beaten body of our Lord, helping Him to stand. The smell of dried blood on the cross probably made him sick. The shouts from the crowd made him cringe. Desperate and uncertain of his fate, he searched the horizon for someone he recognized, someone to help him. There was no one.

The disfigured face of Jesus, bearing a bloodied crown of thorns, turned to him. Our Savior's gentle gaze met Simon's as he pierced through his painful emotions, healing him as they walked together. Christ "was pierced for our offenses and crushed for our iniquity; the punishment that made us whole fell upon him, and by his bruises we have been healed" (Isaiah 53:5).

By accepting the weight of the cross, being yoked with Jesus and united in suffering, Simon's wounds were healed. He was pressed into service to support Jesus, but who was helping whom?

At the end of the journey, they finally arrived at Calvary, and Simon surrendered his grief and struggles to embrace all of his present life, as torturous as it was. He stopped fighting reality. He was illuminated by the Holy One in body and soul, in mind and heart. This walk of redemptive suffering enabled him to transcend his troubles and enter into a radical peace in the presence of Grace Himself. He was now spiritually fortified. He could go on with renewed purpose. He had experienced the Body and Blood of Jesus Christ under the cross.

And so Simon walks home to carry his own cross with love.

This is what we do at every Mass. We take our struggles and surrender them to Jesus as we enter into the radical peace that only He can give through the sacrament of the Eucharist. Over time, our mindset can also be illuminated by Christ. We will "not be conformed to the world, but be transformed by the renewal [our] minds" (Rom 12:2).

We are all Simons, aching from the burdens in our lives—the heartache, the weight gain, the "over-ing," and the chaos of children, family, and elderly parents. Regularly, we are called and compelled to carry our crosses right beside Jesus, our Savior. But, we are human and want to run away from our crosses until we are finally pressed into service. This is called redemptive suffering—suffering with purpose.

We don't seek it out; it's the daily struggle of our present lives. It is only under the cross of Christ that we are permanently transformed. There is nothing that can be done successfully without Him by our side. No, we cannot solve the problem of overeating and overdrinking without Jesus. Only grace will save us.

There is no mobile app or secular diet program that can fix our dilemmas. Learning truthful scientific and theological information is imperative for optimal health, and the supernatural action of Spiritual Fasting is how we apply it. We may feel like we are drowning in diet options, doctor visits, and advice from every source available, but the answer was right here all along: Spiritual Fasting.

It just makes sense. The answers are always found in God.

Spiritual Fasting is a positive and holy approach, an ancient art, that includes both supernatural grace from the sacraments and our own efforts.

In other words, everything you need is found in the Delay and Pray™ method. All it takes is trading the temporary pleasures of sugar, flour, and alcohol for the long-lasting pleasures of a full life—connecting with people and God, getting outdoors, loving, giving, serving, and enjoying the gift of the church. It's not going to be easy. This is a hard trade for so many reasons. But, everything is possible with God.[5]

Let's be honest with ourselves. Sugar, flour, and alcohol have their place but are not helping you on a daily basis. They are just bandages on the wounds of your emotional life. They offer quick comfort today with long-term negative consequences tomorrow. Delaying these addictive substances will help you discover the wounds of your life (instead of covering them) so that they can finally be healed. There is always a reason behind emotional eating and drinking. With Spiritual

Fasting, we can find it and heal it. We can heal others, at the same time.

Soon, you will wonder how it took you so long to discover this blessing.

VIRTUOUS ACTIONS TO CREATE GOOD HABITS

What if your overdrinking and overeating is ultimately a gift because it necessitates the supernatural tool of Spiritual Fasting? What if Spiritual Fasting helps you permanently lose weight and brings you closer to Christ? What if you are being pressed into service right now and yoked right beside Jesus on your life's journey? What if Spiritual Fasting through the Delay and Pray™ method is the answer for you— an offering to God that you have never considered before? What if this discomfort is your ticket to heaven, so that you can be face-to-face with Jesus forever for all eternity?

It is all possible with God.

In the space provided, write a personal letter to the Lord, surrendering to Him through this weight loss journey of Spiritual Fasting. Ask Jesus to be with you every step of the way. Let Him know that you trust Him to send His holy angels to comfort and guide you with the intercession of the Blessed Virgin Mary and all the saints. You have an entire heavenly realm on your side. Asking God for help and trusting in His mercy is the way to successful Spiritual Fasting.

SPIRITUAL FASTING PRAYER

*Temper my desires toward food and alcohol, O Lord,
and turn my focus toward You. Deliver me from the tendency
to go to extremes that strain both body and soul. Fill me with
virtue so that I may strive for saintly diligence and true love of
You. Help me to be content with what I have instead of constantly
seeking more outside of You. May I come to recognize the grace
of moderation that brings both contentment and appreciation.
Let temperance grow in me and lead me to discover all the other
virtues that bring deeper union with You.*

In Your sacred name, I pray. Amen.

CHAPTER 2

Motivation for the Great Experiment

*"Nor does anyone pour new wine into
old wineskins. If he does, the wine will burst the skins,
and then the wine and the skins are both lost. Rather,
new wine is poured into fresh wineskins."*

—Mark 2:22

GET READY FOR THE Great Experiment. I call permanent weight loss through Spiritual Fasting the *Great Experiment* because each person must be willing to go through a trial-and-error process in order to figure out their personalized formula.

Your personalized formula will begin with two motivational goals. These goals will motivate you from the deepest part of your heart. Your two goals will be what inspire you to behave differently. They will help you to invite the new wine of Christ into the old problem of your weight and health. The powerful motivation of these two goals is where your body and soul become "new wineskins" to hold a fresh outpouring of His grace.

While motives are wired into us as human beings, we can choose the goals that motivate us. The two types of motivational goals that are necessary in the Delay and Pray™ method are your spiritual purpose goal and your physical purpose goal.

The first motivational goal is a spiritual purpose goal.

We refer to this as *The Why That Makes You Cry*. This motivational goal would be impossible without God, and it becomes your spiritual purpose for fasting. Your *Why* is the compelling reason that will help you delay sugar, flour, and alcohol to Sundays. Choose something you are passionate about, something you desire enough to fast for. Examples are: bringing your kids back to Mass, resolving health concerns, inviting financial blessings, healing relationships, repairing the state of the nation or church, and so many more. Having a spiritual purpose tied to your actions changes everything. When you direct your weight loss or health goals toward helping others, the suffering becomes redemptive. The suffering of the *delay*, along with the efficacy of the *pray*, will work for you and for those you love. Saint Peter Chrysologus frames this concept well when he writes, "There are three things by which faith stands firm, devotion remains constant, and virtue endures. They are prayer, fasting and mercy. Prayer knocks at the door, fasting obtains, mercy receives."[1]

The second motivational goal is a physical purpose goal.

Think of this motivational goal as your physical purpose for fasting, and it results in optimal health. While you could measure optimal health in several ways (including bloodwork markers and body measurements—and these are advised) the fastest and easiest way is to measure weight loss, using a scale. Don't let the scale scare you! Many people who are stuck in a sugar, flour, and alcohol cycle fear the scale. It is usually because they tie that number to their worth. This is common and comes from the "old wine" of the diet mentality. We have been enslaved for too long, thinking that a certain number is good and other numbers are bad. However, the number on the scale is just a number. We can consider it as a state of health or comfort.

Is there a scale number at which your body would feel more comfortable? Or a number that would help you live a more healthy lifestyle? Is there a number that would help you reduce or eliminate a certain medication (always discuss this with your doctor)? Then choose a goal weight that will help you achieve this state of optimal health—whatever that means to you.

> *The scale simply provides data;*
> *it doesn't measure your worth in*
> *any way. It is also a compass that*
> *lets you know which direction*
> *you are headed.*

Imagine your scale as an impartial calculator that is letting you know how much everything in your body weighs at that moment. The scale simply provides data; it doesn't measure your worth in any way. It is also a compass that lets you know which direction you are headed. It helps you identify the foods that cause weight gain in your particular body. Your scale is there to assist and give you opportunities to course-correct. It is a trial-and-error fact machine that allows you to participate in Spiritual Fasting. It offers an easy way to personalize your journey. You can lose weight slowly over time by gently working with your body and data from the scale to figure out the right foods for you.

If you are willing to think of weight loss as the Great Experiment, during which you will try and fail again and again in order to find what works for your body and soul—then you will be successful. Thinking of the scale as your tool in the Great Experiment is a new and refreshing perspective.

Your scale can be used for you, not against you!

Why change the way you think about the scale? Because everything starts with how you think. Your thoughts are essential to this process because what you seek, you will find.[2]

In John 1:37-38, Jesus notices two disciples following Him. Then He turns around and asks them warmly, "What are you looking for?"

They didn't give Him a clear answer. Like a lot of people, they didn't know what they wanted and needed. Instead of seeking something specific, they were just walking aimlessly behind Jesus. And they missed their opportunity to tell the King of kings—the very One who could have helped them—the hopes and concerns that were overflowing from their hearts.

> *Jesus is waiting for you.*
> *He is really what you have*
> *been looking for.*

What about you? What are *you* looking for?

You may be new to following Him, or you may have walked in His footsteps for many years. No matter the length of your path as a believer, imagine Jesus noticing that you are following Him. Picture Him turning around and asking you, "What are you looking for?"

Would you be able to answer Him? Do you know what you are looking for?

At the end of this chapter, you will have the opportunity to write down your two motivational goals. Then you will support your goals with a commitment to the sacraments.

Jesus is waiting for you. He is really what you have been looking for. If you commit to Mass, adoration, Scripture study, fellowship, and confession, you will not only find Him, you will find your healing. The overeating and overdrinking will fade away over time because you won't be looking for relief anymore.

If Jesus is your ultimate goal, keep in mind that it's not enough to do the spiritual minimum anymore: only going to Sunday Mass and reading the gospel and homily in the morning. You must demand more of yourself so that you will have the supernatural grace to commit to the journey ahead. Within the Delay and Pray™ method, the baseline for attending the sacraments is to add at least one daily Mass and one hour of weekly adoration, along with monthly confession.

Years ago, I started by adding just one extra daily Mass into my week each year until I found myself attending Mass most days of the week. That means it took me almost five years to become a daily Mass participant. Starting slow is fine!

Are you willing to progress slowly to reach your spiritual and physical goals if it means you'll reach them permanently? That's what I did, and the results are amazing. Adding in the sacraments bit by bit is the foundation and the game-changer. The grace that you will gain from this commitment makes everything possible over time.

Of course, it does.

It was Jesus Himself Who said, "For men, this is impossible, but for God all things are possible" (Matt 19:26).

Optimal health may seem like an impossible journey for you, but with God, it will be possible. You will walk every step with Christ. He is under the cross with you. Don't rush your work beside Him. You will be dying little deaths to yourself along the way and will become happier than you've ever been. These little losses are only the deaths of the vices that have kept you in bondage for years.

> *Delay and Pray™ is the currency of your dreams. It will cost you one drink and one donut at a time, traded for meaningful prayer.*

Delay and Pray™ is the currency of your dreams. It will cost you one drink and one donut at a time, traded for meaningful prayer.

By the time you reach your goals, you will be so glad you paid the price.

VIRTUOUS ACTIONS TO CREATE GOOD HABITS

In the space provided, reflect on what you are looking for. What is *The Why That Makes You Cry*? Write the spiritual purpose goal that will motivate you to delay sugar, flour, and alcohol until Sundays while praying for yourself and others.

Then move to your physical purpose goal. What is the weight goal that you can use as a measurement to keep you adjusting your food and alcohol intake until you are able to find just the right personal formula for your body and soul?

And finally, how will you add the sacraments to your weekly schedule?

SPIRITUAL FASTING PRAYER

*Come, Holy Spirit, enlighten my heart to the ways
of God; come into my mind to know the things of God, and into
my very soul, so that all that I do is for the glory of God. Oh, Holy
Spirit of God, I ask you for the gift of fasting, so that I can offer it
as a penance of love, for the sake of my own soul, and for those of
my brothers and sisters in Christ. Help me to understand the grace
You pour out on us through prayer and fasting. Amen.*

—Wayne Weible, *The Medjugorje Fasting Book*[3]

Nikki struggled with sugar. It may have even been an addiction. Around Christmas time, her desire for sugar was the worst. She wanted to eat all the special sweet treats and indulge during the holiday season. She didn't think she had any options other than to just eat what was in front of her.

One day, her cravings were so overpowering, she asked herself, *What would my life look like if I weren't so engulfed by the desire to have sugar all the time?*

Even as the question came to her, she felt that familiar resistance. She didn't want to give up the comfort of sugar. Life was hard enough, and she didn't want to add even more difficulty.

Then Nikki heard about the Delay and Pray™ Group Coaching Experience. It gave her hope to know there were some tools to help her navigate seasons like Christmas and Easter, when it was difficult to eat with calm restraint.

So Nikki joined Delay and Pray™ even though she didn't have a huge weight goal in mind. She was attracted by the testimonials from clients, as well as the spiritual component. She really liked that her sacrifices wouldn't be just for her, but would also be to help the family members for whom she was praying.

Nikki was nervous as the program started, but she saw that everybody was just like her. The other women were at different weights, and everyone was just trying to figure it out. She felt a sense of connection and community right away. The simplicity of the program surprised her, and the opportunity to go through the experience with others felt exciting.

I think I'm in the right place now, she remembers thinking. *I'm among people who are also trying their very best. I'll be okay here.*

She started to love how the group really holds the space for women to get coached and talk about topics that are deeply sensitive. "Even if I ate off protocol earlier in the day, the reminder of Spiritual Fasting on the coaching call would really hone in on my desires for sugar, flour, and alcohol and remind me that this is making a difference—it is worth something. Sometimes the reminder came through a miracle that happened or someone in the group who really needed extra prayer and fasting," she said.

By the end of the program, Nikki no longer desired the things she used to. Her sugar cravings tapered down, and for the most part, she was able to go Monday through Saturday without any huge cravings.

Her focus has permanently shifted, too. She's lost some weight and likes how she fits into her clothes, but what she likes even more is how she looks in pictures. She feels better about her body and herself. She is empowered to make good choices about food. When there's a dessert table, she makes a conscious decision about what she's eating.

Nikki's favorite result is how her personal transformation has strengthened her marriage. Her husband does little things to support her new lifestyle, and recently she noticed that she called his gestures "really sweet."

She laughs at the irony.

"It's funny I used the word sweet because I struggled so much with sugar before the program, but this is a sweetness I can really savor, you know?"

CHAPTER 3

Happy, Thin, and Rich Right Now

"May the peace of the Lord be with you always, because when you possess peace every day you will be truly rich."

—Blessed Pier Giorgio Frassati[1]

WHEN IT COMES TO motivational goals, many people say they just wish they were happy, thin, and rich. They think if they ever arrived at that fantasy destination, there would be no more problems, and life would become easier. They imagine that they would finally experience a peaceful heart. But the truth is that peace must come before anything else. You already have access to a peace that is beyond all understanding.[2]

In other words, you can be happy, thin, and rich right now.

You were created by God to be blessed and prosperous. You were made to be happy as a child of God, healthy in body and soul, and rich in mercy and kindness. These are the spiritual things that will bring you peace right now. The physical goals will follow. As Blessed Pier Giorgio states, "If you possess peace every day, you will be truly rich."[3]

So how do we possess peace?

It comes down to our nature and the knowledge of what is making us unhappy. When God created Adam and Eve, He gave them three gifts that were for all of us:[4]

The first gift was human dignity. We are all made in His image and likeness with both a body and a soul that are integrated. Within this body-and-soul composite, humans received a mind and a will, having certain natural drives and needs. Everything that God created for and within Adam and Eve was good.

> At the Fall of Man, we lost the gift of sanctifying grace that was infused at conception, as well as the coordinating gift of integrity that ordered our passions from birth. Now we have to work at ordering our passions.

The second gift was integrity. Integrity made it easy to keep their drives and passions in perfect order. It was easy to be good! Oh, if this were still true for us now. For Adam and Eve, the flesh was docile to the Holy Spirit. This is how we were supposed to be.

The third gift was sanctifying grace. This grace is a portion of

God's own life, and it opens the human soul to the vision of God for eternal life.

But Adam and Eve were tempted by the devil, and they sinned. Their sin opened our flesh to disordered reason and rebellion. At the Fall of Man, we lost the gift of sanctifying grace that was infused at conception, as well as the coordinating gift of integrity that ordered our passions from birth. Now we have to work at ordering our passions. We are still blessed with the gift of human dignity, but we need to take the hand of Jesus to again receive integrity and sanctifying grace to work out our salvation until heaven.

Can you begin to see why you may not be happy automatically or access peace easily? While we are on this earth, our best life will require intention. Don't feel badly if you experience rebellious thoughts or emotions at times. Give yourself compassion and learn to lean into the sacraments and a deep relationship with God.

The *Catechism of the Catholic Church* defines sanctifying grace this way:

> Sanctifying grace is the gratuitous gift of His life that God makes to us; it is infused by the Holy Spirit into the soul to heal it of sin and to sanctify it. Sanctifying grace makes us "pleasing to God." Charisms, special graces of the Holy Spirit, are oriented to sanctifying grace and are intended for the common good of the Church. God also acts through many actual graces, to be distinguished from habitual grace which is permanent in us (CCC 2023-2024).[4]

Through Baptism, the Holy Trinity comes to dwell in our hearts, whether we are babies or adults. The gift that returns with that indwelling of the Spirit is sanctifying grace. The life of God, through the Holy Spirit, enters the human soul, and everything changes. This is why Baptism is essential. It is the first step to peace.

With sanctifying grace, we fuel our minds, or intellect, with Truth so that we can direct our free will to make the decisions that are for our highest good. It is up to us to take authority over our minds by managing our thoughts and emotions. Overeating and overdrinking are often symptoms of a mind gone wild. Examining your thoughts is imperative to living the life you were meant to live. Spiritual Fasting by delaying sugar, flour, and alcohol to Sundays or feast days is only possible by inviting God's sanctifying grace into our minds.

Let's face it, a lack of grace results in a darkening of the intellect and a weakening of the will. As St. Paul exhorts, "For I do not do the good I want, but I do the evil I do not want. Now if I do what I do not want, it is no longer I who do it, but sin that dwells in me" (Rom 7:19-20).

> *Believing you are happy, thin, and rich right now isn't just toxic positivity. Problems will always be with you, but you can steady yourself with God amidst the chaos of daily living.*

St. Pope John Paul II also emphasizes the importance of sanctifying grace, saying, "'It is evident that original sin in Adam's descendants has not the character of personal guilt. It is the privation of sanctifying grace...' Privation really means a lack of what ought to be there. So when we speak of being born without sanctifying grace (original sin) by birth, it would be more accurate to speak of the non-transmission of sanctifying grace."[5]

Sometimes we look at food and alcohol as if these choices are beyond our control. But through God's sanctifying grace, we can manage our bodies and souls. Don't let your mind go wild. Learn about yourself and what God has in store for your life. Seek to understand your body-and-soul composite as a human being. Through God and our individual agency, we can stay in a state of grace so that we can manage our minds ... right up to the moment this earthly life is over.

Believing you are happy, thin, and rich right now isn't just toxic positivity. Problems will always be with you, but you can steady yourself with God amidst the chaos of daily living. Then you can attain the life of your dreams here on earth. This happens spiritually first, then physically.

Until now, Jesus may have been the missing piece in your health. But, don't confuse running to Him as something that will be easy. You are going to have to show up and do quite a bit of work. The Lord promised that labor would be part of a good life when He said, "'The harvest is abundant, but the laborers are few. Therefore, ask the Lord of the harvest to send out laborers for his harvest" (Matt 9:37-38).

So while you wait for your personal harvest, enjoy the process. Put a beautiful outfit on that precious body of yours. Clean up your living space, look around, and love it. Take stock of your bank accounts and give thanks for what you have right now. Start being a lover and a giver. Express gratitude for all the blessings you already have, and then get ready—your dreams are about to explode!

I'm going to teach you how to think about the present in order to harness the future, as God wants us to do. He loves to work in the realm of impossibility. You can move toward the impossible, even if you are feeling some doubt. When Jesus's disciples doubted, He told them, "For men this is impossible, but for God all things are possible" (Matt 19:26). You are headed for the Promised Land, friend. The goals you are setting will motivate you to do the work required to get there.

In my studies at The Life Coach School, a memorable phrase came up again and again: *Life is always 50% happy and 50% crappy.* Though that might sound a bit crude, the rhyme makes this truth easy to remember. No one encounters a lifetime of flawless circumstances. There will be good and bad days. But both the happy and the crappy are so much better when you engage the suffering without numbing yourself through "over-ing."

So. Much. Better.

> Sure, I have had to learn
> how to seek all that was true,
> good, and beautiful. But the
> more I keep seeking it,
> the more I keep finding it.

If you can learn to enjoy your life as it is now and offer up your suffering to Jesus, then you will become transformed in Christ and help others at the same time. Christ-centered people are happy, thin, and rich in their minds because they possess God, are grateful for the present, and know their mission before Him. When they already have the peace they need today, then there is no hurry to arrive at a fantasy future.

I'm happy, thin, and rich right now. I say that as I write this book in an old lake house that one day will be renovated. We just bought it, and it is beautiful in my mind. That's how I think of it on purpose.

It is a dream come true, a work in progress. I love this old creaky house right now, even though I also envision what it will become. Living here has taught me to be patient and trust God in all things. It has taught me to enjoy where I am right now. The imperfections of this lake house are simply an opportunity for growth. The same perspective is available to me when I think about my body. I already see myself as happy, thin, and rich. This is my gorgeous life, and I love it.

Sure, I have had to learn how to seek all that is true, good, and beautiful. But the more I keep seeking it, the more I keep finding it. I have stopped looking for my limitations and started paying attention to my dreams. I thank God ahead of time, praying Scripture over every part of my day. I believe that God can do what I can't, and I mount up evidence in favor of what He wants for me.

How do I do this?

Humility isn't purchased, but it does come at a great cost.

I am willing to write goals down and miss the mark. Yes, you read that right. I am willing to miss my goals as well as meet them. Every time I fail, I evaluate and try again. In doing so, I have developed resilience. Every part of my goal process goes on paper, including my food regimen and personal reflections. Most of all, I decide it's okay for me to fail.

That decision was put to the test when I decided to announce to the world that I was The Catholic Fasting Coach. Those closest to me had a front row seat to watch me fail in fasting again and again, as I indulged in alcohol and the occasional slice of pizza during the week.

But I tried it the next week and the next until I succeeded.

Humility isn't purchased, but it does come at a great cost.

So, my question to you is how hard are you willing to try to get this done? Are you willing to get under that cross with Jesus? Are you willing to change your beliefs about what is possible? To accept the reality that Spiritual Fasting is for you and not against you?

Let's be honest, it's not fun under the cross. I originally crawled under there for me, begging to be transformed; now I'm under there for the sheer love of Him. There is no finish line that I can see. There is no "wagon" to fall off of. You and I will be transforming from glory to glory[6] every day for the rest of our lives.

In 2 Corinthians 12:9, Paul brings God his weaknesses, and God tells him that His "power is made perfect in weakness." For that reason, Paul boasts about his weaknesses from then on.

> *There is no "wagon" to fall off of.*
> *You and I will be transforming*
> *from glory to glory every day*
> *for the rest of our lives.*

God's power is made perfect in my weaknesses, too. For that reason, I am so thankful for the overeating and overdrinking struggles that make me feel weak. I boast of my weaknesses because they have brought me to Him.

I am no longer ashamed. God has entered into all of that shame and is healing it minute by minute. Anything good that I do is because of God's glory. All the rest is just me working out my salvation here on earth. This transformation makes me feel happy, thin, and rich.

And, free.

You have to go through the discomfort of the cross to get to the transformation. As Fr. Chad Ripperger says, "The only way to delight is through mortification."[7]

So, what delights you? What does *happy* mean to you? What do *thin* and *rich* mean to you? Those words can be defined by your imagination with the guidance of Scripture and the Holy Spirit.

God has given us an amazing imagination that drives our emotions. We can literally generate emotions with our imagination through images, music, reading, writing, storytelling, daydreaming, watching movies, and even through adoration. Our imagination helps us to build curiosity and ignite the motivation of what is possible in our lives.

What we desire to achieve, we first need to envision. Then we can work toward that dream in the form of visualized goals. Having a clear vision helps us endure the suffering that will occur along the way, as we reach every goal over time.

In this book, we will concentrate on creating happiness right now regardless of weight or health. And, we will become wealthy in spirit as we grow in love and compassion for ourselves and others. This is the only way out of "over-ing." You get to decide to love yourself as God loves you and stop shaming yourself into being different. It is in this frame of mind that will enable you to pray and fast yourself into your dreams.

All while praying and fasting others into their dreams, too.

VIRTUOUS ACTIONS TO CREATE GOOD HABITS

In the space provided:

1. Write out clear definitions of what the words *happy*, *thin*, and *rich* mean to you. Be honest, your definitions may be broken, worldly, or even selfish. But, if you bring them before Jesus, He will help you with your desires. He longs for you to speak to Him and wrestle with Him about your dreams. Let the Lord transform your desires from weight loss to holiness, from rich in money to rich in mercy, and from happiness due to worldly pleasure to happiness with Him.

2. What do you think the Lord desires for you in these areas?

_____

_____

_____

_____

_____

_____

_____

_____

_____

_____

_____

_____

_____

_____

3. Activate your imagination and describe a future scene where you are enjoying what it feels like to be all three.

_____

_____

_____

_____

_____

_____

_____

SPIRITUAL FASTING PRAYER

*Oh, Holy Spirit, on this day, I resolve to fast as Our Lady asks
of me. I have decided to fast because your prophets fasted. I am
fasting because Jesus, my Lord, fasted. I am fasting, so that I can be
a true disciple and true apostle and a true daughter/son of Mary.
I present this day of fasting to You, so that I listen to Your Word,
I become You to those around me, and I see them as You. Help me,
Holy Spirit, to fast with my heart.*

—Wayne Weible, *The Medjugorje Fasting Book*[8]

CHAPTER 4

Believing Harder Than You Work

"I do believe. Help my unbelief."
—Mark 9:24

IN SEPTEMBER OF 2020, the Covid Pandemic had been in full swing for six months and was wreaking havoc on the whole world. My Mom was 90 years old and living in a retirement home just a couple miles down the road. I am her last child of eight kids, and we have always been the best of friends. One of my siblings or I visited her almost every day of the week. We had cared for our mom for the last 25 years since our father had died. My mom was typically funny, loving, giving, and wonderful to be around.

When the lockdown started in March, we were not allowed inside the facility so we had a little party under her window for her

91st birthday. We never dreamed the restrictions would last but a few weeks. Yet, the weeks dragged on. After six months of dropping off meals and talking by phone under her window, she began crying whenever we talked, and we contemplated taking her out of the facility to live with one of us. She just couldn't bear being locked away by herself anymore. We were beside ourselves about what to do.

Even with occasional visits to the lobby, Mom started to decline. She fell quite a bit and was hallucinating. Her health became complicated. Our family began feuding over what was best for her, and all of us felt fear, anger, sadness, and despair about the situation. We prayed and had family meetings to try and figure it out.

My sugar, flour, and alcohol consumption was at an all-time high as I ate my way through the emotional roller coaster. At one point, I was so upset by trying to get my Mom into a better situation that I contemplated putting a ladder in my car and crawling into her window on the second floor. My sister pleaded with me not to do this; she worried that I would get arrested. But that was how desperate I felt! I reconsidered the "ladder rescue plan," hung up the phone, and dropped to my knees in prayer.

It was at this very moment that I was led to start fasting for the situation.

God was calling me to Spiritually Fast—there was no other option to help my mom. I had tried Spiritual Fasting so many times in the last 20 years, failing every time. Dieting was like an unintended hobby of mine, and weight loss took much of my mental and physical energy. But at that moment of crisis, I realized that I finally had the spiritual purpose I needed to make this happen. I decided to combine prayer and the delay of sugar, flour, and alcohol from my diet to enable me to go without food for longer periods of time.

After experimenting with different regimens and amping up my reception of the sacraments to receive all the grace possible—I was able to pray and fast for the breakthrough of getting to come inside the retirement home to care for my mom. After Spiritual Fasting for a short time (about three weeks), we were finally able to enter the retirement home where we cared for our mom 24/7. She died peacefully a few months later. We were all by her side that day. As far as we could see, we were the only ones allowed in the building at that time. It was a true miracle.

And it wouldn't have been possible without belief.

Please understand that the miracle of being able to care for my mother did not come about because of any hard work that my siblings or I did. We did not protest outside the building. We did not call higher and more important people in the company. We did not contact the local newspaper or television station, either. No, the miracle happened as a result of prayer and fasting, and those humble actions are only made possible by the fuel of belief in God's mighty power.

The belief that God can heal you and help you reach your goals is an important part of the Great Experiment. It is in the act of believing that you will discover how you became attached to overeating and overdrinking. Somewhere along the line, you became dependent on it to flatten the ups and downs of your life. And the reason why diets have failed in the past is because they were only about changing the food, not the belief behind the food.

Do you know what you believe about food? Have you ever thought about it, ever tried to figure it out? If we don't crawl under the cross beside Jesus to figure ourselves out with Him, then we will continue to subconsciously fight for our limiting beliefs. Somewhere in our subconscious minds we have become resigned to them. Those beliefs may be habitual thoughts now, but they can be broken. Through Spiritual Fasting, even vices can be turned into virtues.

What is a belief? In simple terms, beliefs are thoughts that you think over and over again until they become part of you. As a Catholic, we recite the Nicene Creed at the beginning of every Mass. I have recited this prayer for 50 years, and I believe it. It is a tenet of the Catholic faith and a unity prayer for all of us to say "yes" to. I have prayed it so many times that I've memorized it. I believe it more and more every day as I grow older.

> *In simple terms, beliefs are thoughts that you think over and over again until they become part of you.*

Sometimes we do the same thing when we encounter ideas that are not good to believe. The diet mentality filled with thoughts that you have recited over and over since childhood is not helpful. Thoughts like "I am only worthy if I weigh X," or "When I'm thin, I will be happy," or "I'm out of control with my weight—as usual," or "Losing weight is impossible," are beliefs that can become memorized habits in our thought life.

We beat ourselves up with these thoughts, and over time, we don't even know we are thinking them anymore. They are patterns that are hard to interrupt. If we fight for them, even subconsciously, we'll prove them true 100 percent of the time. This is why we need to believe in God's promise of healing through redemption so strongly.

Belief in Truth is the only hope of transformation.

In her book *Women, Food, and God*, Geneen Roth writes, "The shape of your body obeys the shape of your beliefs about love, value, and possibility. To change your body, you must first understand that which is shaping it" (p.79).[1]

What happens if you choose to change the shape of your beliefs? What if you wake up and start the day fresh with a *Nunc Coepi* type of attitude? Don't leave the Nicene Creed just for Sundays. Say parts of it every morning as you get out of bed: *I believe in God, the Father Almighty, Maker of heaven and earth—and He and I have work to do today. I am thin in body, rich in mercy, and ready to go!*

> *Your body and bank account*
> *will follow your beliefs.*

Your body and bank account will follow your beliefs. Together, you and God can do something about your weight, your job, and your health. Believe it. When you want to shift your beliefs, Scripture is a great start because it is Truth. I pray it, say it, and memorize it. I build new habits and patterns into my subconscious mind. I intentionally think thoughts like, *I am a person who delays sugar, flour, and alcohol to Sundays.* I say it over and over and over again until it starts to come true—even after many failures. As soon as I see the change happening, I reflect on it in my thought: *Thank you God, that I am a person who delays sugar, flour, and alcohol to Sundays.* It took me a while to realize that He is the one that is transforming me. He deserves thanksgiving. His thoughts are way above my thoughts.[2]

I have to admit: For a long time, my thoughts stayed on sugar, flour, and alcohol.

Spiritual Fasting helps us identify our attachments to certain things. Eventually, sugar and flour took a back seat for me, but alcohol was the last to move. Because my thoughts stayed on alcohol, it became one of my comfortable attachments. Alcohol is a lifestyle for our family. Most of our social interactions involve some type of liquor and food—a dinner reservation over a craft beer with a catchy name or a nice glass of wine in front of a roaring fireplace in the winter. Seems innocent enough. But for me, alcohol was even harder to delay than sugar and flour. Alcohol felt so different. It was tripping me up. I was constantly trying to find a way to keep drinking, instead of trying to find a way to stop drinking. It was as if I were saying to the Lord, "I'm not sure if I will it. But, would You please do it anyway? Would You just take care of this alcohol attachment against my will?"

> *You don't realize how attached you are to sugar, flour, alcohol, and even processed food, until you decide to delay them.*

No, He's not going to do that because He has given us free will.

I didn't notice my unwillingness to detach from alcohol until after a year of semi-successfully delaying alcohol for different periods of time. You don't realize how attached you are to sugar, flour, alcohol, and even processed food, until you decide to delay them. You and I are going to need God's help to do it. As Jesus says in John 5:19, "Amen, amen, I say to you, the Son can do nothing by himself; he can do only what he sees the Father doing."

Even Jesus understands that He can do nothing without the Father. The same is true for us. When we enter into Spiritual Fasting, we face the fact that we don't want to detach from temporary comforts.

One year, I was proud of myself for fasting from sugar, flour, and alcohol for the sanctity of life in January. What I didn't realize back then, is that deep down in my unconscious beliefs, I knew I could pick up drinking again in February before embarking on another dry season during Lent. But, when those specific times of fasting came to an end, I was back to regularly negotiating with myself about alcohol: *How about I add a glass of wine for dinner on Tuesday or maybe Thursday. That's not bad. It will help me get to Friday night.* And, then when I arrived at Friday night, which I had purposed to be free of alcohol, I'd think: *I'll just have one instead of two.*

Be aware that I did not binge or drink heavily at all—just a couple glasses of wine or a few hard seltzers. But Jesus was asking, "Why drink during the week at all?" For some reason, I could not delay drinking on Friday nights, the most important penitential fasting day of the week in the Catholic Church outside of Lent.

Wednesdays and Fridays are fasting days in the Catholic Church because these are the days that are before and after the Institution of the Eucharist that occurred on Holy Thursday. So, in commemoration of that beautiful day, the Blessed Mother asks that we fast. In the Delay and Pray™ method, we abstain from meat along with the sugar, flour, and alcohol on Wednesdays and Fridays.

Well, Fridays have always been a day of celebration in my mind. It felt like the party day to enjoy the end of the week by going out to eat or ordering in pizza, to have a beer or glass of wine (or two or three), and to relax with all of my attachments: sugar, flour, and alcohol. I didn't want my Fridays to change, but I knew *I* needed to change. So meat was the first thing I decided to give up. Later, I gave up sugar and flour—but alcohol? Now *that* was a difficult sacrifice. At first, I would have thoughts such as, *I'll switch Friday for Thursday when it comes to alcohol, or I'll fast from 5pm Thursday to 5pm Friday.* I was making so many excuses and justifying every possible way I could drink alcohol on Friday nights.

I always work with a life coach to reach my goals. At the time, my coach asked me why I believed that Fridays were for drinking alcohol. My answer was because that is how I grew up and how I lived my life, and I didn't want to change that. Fridays were for fun and without alcohol, how could they be fun?

Thoughts reveal your deeply held beliefs, and mine was: *Friday nights are for drinking and fun.*

This was a limiting belief that I was choosing to the detriment of my goals. Due to continually thinking this thought, I was making sure I believed it 100 percent. Thoughts always end up in your results if you don't change them, so the result was that I was drinking on Friday nights in anguish, almost against my will. This wasn't fun at all!

Even thinking of sacrificing for others just made me feel guilty and was not enough to help me break the attachment or addiction to the Friday night buzz. I had a hard time even reframing it into sacrifice. We coached on this for weeks.

Finally she said, "Okay great. You won't change it then."

Ugh. That was not the answer that I was looking for.

I realized right then that I did not believe that I could have a sober Friday night and still have fun, therefore it wouldn't even begin to happen. So, instead of tackling a new set of actions, I started to tackle the belief.

I decided to figure this out every week with my rosary while in front of Jesus in the Blessed Sacrament. He let me know that the alcohol was an idol, an attachment standing between us. I wasn't constantly taking my attachment to alcohol into the gaze of Jesus week after week. I thought a visit every now and then would be enough. No, it would take an all-out assault by all the sacraments to cut this thread that was holding me back. I began telling myself, "I believe I can stop drinking on Fridays. I am a person who fasts for others on Fridays. 'For God all things are possible.'"[3]

I chose a *Why That Makes Me Cry* to fast for and set out on the Great Experiment to figure out myself with Jesus. I ordered books on the effects of alcohol and how to stop. I read testimonials of alcoholics who had stopped drinking and how their lives were so much better. I found all this information fascinating. Although I wasn't a classic alcoholic, I really was addicted to alcohol on that one night every week. I waited for alcohol, anticipated alcohol, and longed for alcohol.

And, then one day, I stopped it.

I was able to do so because I had fueled my intellect with the truth of what alcohol was doing to my body. I recognized that I wanted a way to escape the work week and start the weekend with the "enjoyment" of a buzz. I took the problem to adoration and planned not to drink on Friday nights. I followed my own program, getting coached on the subject, giving myself permission to fail as much as possible to succeed, and repeating the belief ahead of time: "I do not drink on Friday nights," and "I delay alcohol on Friday nights," and "Friday nights are for delaying and praying." Also, I worked on a strategy of going to the sacraments as often as possible, staying busy, exercising, praying, substituting non-alcoholic beverages, and managing my mind. Finally, I started to pray very hard for people who struggle with alcohol in general.

At first, Friday nights were not fun.

Eventually, I noticed the urge to have a drink would come, and it would go. The more I allowed myself to feel the urge and not feed the urge, the easier it became to let it go. I delayed and prayed over and over. It became easier and easier. Those nights are so wrapped in redemptive suffering now that they are actually fun in a different and better way. I am continuously praying and fasting for so many people on Friday nights. The urge for a drink hasn't completely gone away, but it is manageable and reminds me to pray. This must be what the saints mean when they thank God for the struggle.

> *Belief has been*
> *transformational for me.*
> *And it will be for you, too.*

I still drink on Saturday nights and occasionally on Sundays, and my passions are rightly ordered. This is what Spiritual Fasting does for us. It forces us to take a look at our beliefs and the lies we are telling ourselves. It helps us trade vices for virtues. It is a challenge, but if you believe, you can do it.

Belief has been transformational for me. And it will be for you, too.

VIRTUOUS ACTIONS TO CREATE GOOD HABITS

In the space provided, write your reflection on the following questions. What repeating thoughts have become beliefs for you? How are your beliefs shaping your body? Are you able to love, value, and believe the impossible right now?

SPIRITUAL FASTING PRAYER

Mary, you were free in your heart and bound to nothing except the Father's will. Obtain by prayer the grace of a joyful fast for me today in which my heart will be able to sing with you a thanksgiving song. Through this fast cleanse me of all bad habits and calm down my passions, and let your virtues increase in me. Let the depth of my soul open to your grace through this fast so that it may totally affect and cleanse me.

—Fr. Slavko Barbaric, *Pray With The Heart!*[4]

Jackie was a Catholic who had been away from the Church for about 25 years. She was 30 pounds overweight, and had started looking for answers. That's when she stumbled upon a podcast episode where Beth was being interviewed, and Jackie thought to herself, *Gosh! I could do that! That's not a diet; it's something entirely different.*

It struck her that Spiritual Fasting is a real change from dieting. The orderly framework of the program also resonated with Jackie, who is a very structured person and a statistician by trade. She started listening to all of Beth's podcasts and trying her own version of Spiritual Fasting to see if she could really do it. She was surprised by how her prayer life deepened and her connection with God grew so quickly. She decided to join the Delay and Pray ™ program.

During Lent that year, she absentmindedly left a Stations of the Cross booklet on the counter, and her husband, who was raised Baptist but had been engaging in New Age practices and wouldn't step foot into a church, began flipping through the booklet. While she was gone on a business trip, he ordered wooden Stations of the Cross, built foundations for each station, and placed them on their four-acre property. She was surprised and delighted to see them when she returned home, and now every Saturday morning she goes out to pray at the Stations of the Cross.

Eventually, her husband started coming to Church with her and becoming friends with people at the parish. Recently, he shared that he wants to convert to Catholicism. He'll start

RCIA soon, and the two are now focused on helping each other get to heaven.

When Jackie started the program, she was praying for 28 different miracles, and 26 have come to pass. One of the biggest miracles is something that wasn't on her original list. When a massive hurricane hit her state of Florida, it knocked down dozens of trees on her property. But the Stations of the Cross that her husband had installed remained untouched, although broken branches and debris fell all around them.

Jackie emphasizes that while she's lost 25 pounds, that's secondary to the emotional and spiritual benefit and the miracles she's seen. She had broken relationships with people that she hadn't seen for years, but God has given her unexpected opportunities. She even joined a family reunion, reconnecting with six or seven people there. Now their relationships are loving, warm, and even welcome hugs.

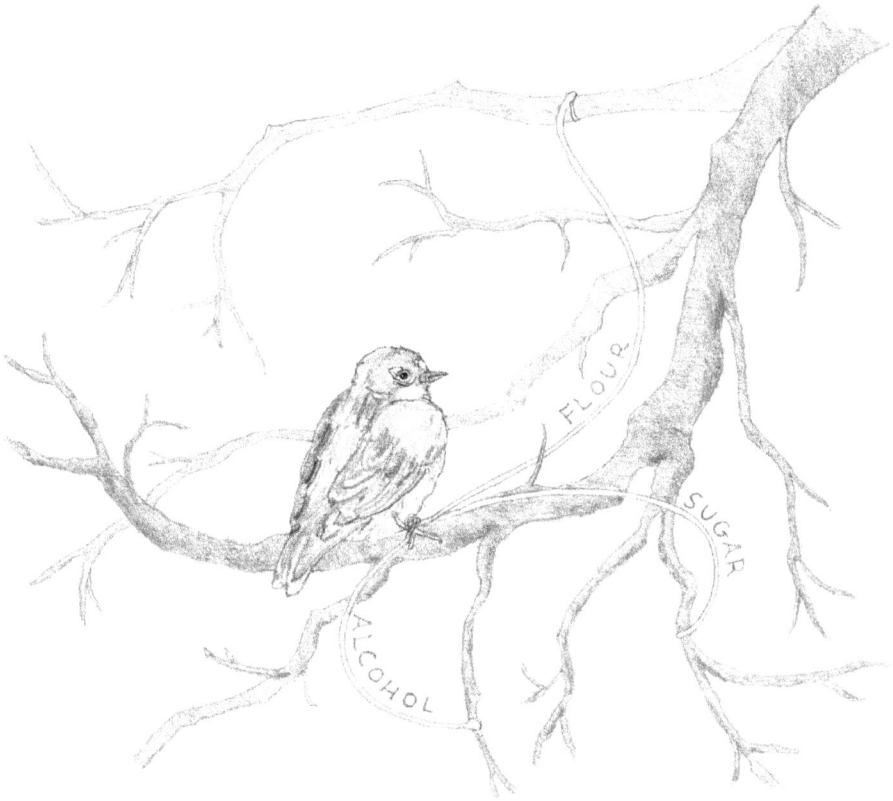

Cut the strings of sugar, flour, and alcohol that tie you down.
You were made to fly.

CHAPTER 5

The Thought Model of Possibility with God

"Be transformed by the renewal of your minds."
—Romans 12:2

BECAUSE OUR THOUGHTS BECOME our beliefs, they are critical to permanent weight loss and Spiritual Fasting. What we think and believe determine how we show up in the world. In that way, our thought patterns are moving us closer to or further away from our goals.

Weight loss just for the sake of vanity is entirely self-focused. However, we can choose a new mindset that helps us to be more

God-focused and other-focused. You will be amazed how much faster desirable results come when the labor is done in love for our neighbor or a larger spiritual purpose. An unselfish mindset changes us. In the church document Gaudium et Spes we read that "man cannot fully find himself except through a sincere gift of himself."[1]

> *What we think and believe determine how we show up in the world. In that way, our thought patterns are moving us closer to or further away from our goals.*

What was once a harried diet mindset is transformed into an intentional life of living for others. It is no longer about your limitations, but about the abundance that you have to give. Delaying sugar, flour, and alcohol to Sundays for a higher purpose will require deliberate thought-shifts to stay on course. You can't consider weight loss without considering your soul, and you can't consider Spiritual Fasting without considering your body. They are integrated from head to toe.

When we purposefully think about our thinking, aligning it with God's will, we can shift our thoughts for the better. Eventually, that changes our behavior. This is how we find ourselves and our God-given mission. If a thought-shift feels forced at first, you can add a smaller thought-shift in-between. For example, many new clients come to me with the thought, "I am not enough." It isn't easy for them to shift directly to "I am more than enough." That's when I show them that they can create a bridge thought. "I am not enough" can shift to "God has equipped me with more than enough," which eventually shifts to "I am more than enough." When you interject the powerful name of God into the thought, He will give you a different view of the circumstances you are experiencing in your life. His view will always serve your highest good. The circumstance doesn't even have to change as long as your thoughts about it do.

Thought-shifts will always result in emotion-shifts.

Consider that first thought: "I am not enough."

When you think this, what feeling does it give you? A negative thought like this one can lead to a feeling of despair or shame. Whatever the feeling is, it usually comes from a place of lack or deprivation. The feeling itself causes physical discomfort in mind and body. It is called a *feeling* because it is a cascade of chemicals in your body that you can literally feel as a sensation.

> *Thought-shifts will always*
> *result in emotion-shifts.*

That feeling drives an action or inaction. The actions that proceed from despair could be ruminating on the situation or eating the rest of the donuts in the box. The inactions that proceed from shame could be not calling a friend for support or not journaling for days at a time. These behaviors that you do (or fail to do) don't work in your favor.

Now, let's look at the thought-shift: "I am more than enough with God."

This thought may elicit a feeling of peace or bold confidence. The actions that proceed from peace could be taking a deep breath, saying a Rosary, reading Scripture, or going for a walk. The inactions that proceed from bold confidence could be turning away from food that is not planned for today or taking a break to let your mind rest for a while. These are all options when the urges and cravings come.

You always have the option to choose what to think in the moment of craving. Work on choosing a thought that brings great results. Then, practice, practice, practice it. You will fail a lot at first, but there are fruits from the good thoughts that we think, and over time you will succeed and shape your body accordingly.

> *You always have the option to choose what to think in the moment of craving. Work on choosing a thought that brings great results.*

Do you see how powerful your mind is? Your thinking drives the chemical cascade of your emotions for better or worse. Thoughts that include trusting God and blessing the situation for everyone involved will produce strong positive feelings and better behavior with the vital assistance of the Holy Spirit and grace. If you fail several times before you can shift, then you are normal and not broken. It takes time, discomfort, and patience to build new neural pathways in your brain. Your mind is deeply in need of self-management and being renewed by Christ. Your mind can tell you lies, and it can tell you truths. Jesus will help you discern between the two through prayer, Scripture, sacraments, and using a wonderful tool called a Thought Model.

A Thought Model is a practical framework that helps you assess and address your thoughts. Saint Thomas Aquinas first explained this model when he devised the concept of the Ontological Man. It has since been revised into an easy formula to understand and apply. In a nutshell, it goes like this:

Thoughts cause Feelings cause Actions cause Results.

This predictable cycle reveals how your thoughts result in consequences for your soul. What we do here on earth affects our entrance into Heaven. And it all starts with thoughts.

Consider the Penitential Act that we recite at Mass. It states:

I confess to almighty God and to you, my brothers and sisters, that I have greatly sinned through my thoughts and in my words, in what I have done, and in what I have failed to do; through my fault, through my fault, through my most grievous fault; therefore I ask blessed Mary ever-Virgin, all the angels and saints, and you, my brothers and sisters, to pray for me to the Lord our God.

It is interesting that during this Act we tap our chest where our heart is and recite three times: "Through my fault, through my fault, through my most grievous fault." It is as if we are using our body to wake up our soul, saying, "Hey! Wake up! What thoughts are stopping you from reaching the dreams and mission that God has written on your heart? What thoughts are causing you to yell at your spouse or your children?"

Have you ever wondered why we say we "greatly sin in our thoughts?" Because we get to choose them. This is our free will. Thoughts don't just happen to us; we can actually choose what we think about. And, those thoughts eventually will burst out as words. All too often, they are words we don't even mean! Thank God for confession and for Catholic mindset coaching where I am learning to do this less and less. You and I can become virtuous through paying close attention to our minds with a Thought Model. Learning to shift your thoughts will bring about miracles for you. It has for me.

A few years ago, my husband and I were searching for a lake house to buy, but we couldn't find one in our price range that was even nice enough to use for the summers. We searched for two years around our area without any luck.

> *Learning to shift your thoughts*
> *will bring about miracles for you.*

At one point, I noticed in my journal that my thoughts were very negative:

"Maybe we just don't have enough money to buy a lake house."

"These houses and prices are awful!"

"This will never work."

There it is, right there. That thought was going to produce certain results. If I continued to think that buying a lake house would never work, then it probably wouldn't work. I was creating the reality of not finding a good property with my negative thoughts, appearing as words on the paper. Had I not done the important work of shifting those thoughts, we probably wouldn't have found the home of our dreams.

How did I do it? I invited Jesus into those thoughts with Spiritual Fasting. I had been praying for Him to find us a house, but I hadn't intentionally chosen my thoughts or fasted for it. So I wrote down the intention on my prayer and fasting list, prayed diligently for a breakthrough, and started to delay sugar, flour, and alcohol for the perfect house to buy. I also held my goal with "loose hands" and let Jesus know this was all His decision. If He didn't want us to buy a lake house then I was okay with Him closing the door on this dream and directing me to another. This simple shift immediately felt lighter and more positive.

The fasting caused me to look outward in the situation because that is what fasting does. It transforms us from self-centered to others-centered. I began thinking, "How can I help others in this situation?" I focused on blessing others by fasting and prayers like this one:

> "Lord, please help us to find the perfect lake house to entertain our family and friends. May our purchase bless the owner of that home in many ways. Let our money be of great blessing to all involved. Help us to be prudent yet generous in our offer. Let this home be filled with enduring love and gratitude. May it be a place of warmth where You will make Your dwelling with us forever. Amen."

The more I prayed and fasted, the more my thought-shift became my new belief: "The lake house is coming. It is beautiful and will be a blessing to all."

I asked Jesus how we could bless someone else with our current home if we were to purchase a year-round lake house. I started to re-paint and prepare it inside and out to be sold to a beautiful family who would love it and raise their children in it, as we had done. Before I ever met them, I fasted for the family who would buy our house and the family we would buy from. I expected a miracle.

The results were indeed miraculous.

One wintry day we drove over to an open house to see a small lake house that was for sale. It was there that we met Theresa, who was also looking for a new home herself. She was crying as she viewed the house, and we asked her if she was okay. Her emotions were high because just months before, she had lost her husband in her current house and was looking to move out as soon as possible. We listened and talked with her until we left an hour later without putting an offer on the house. We didn't expect to see Theresa again.

The next day, Theresa called our realtor and asked if we wanted to look at her current house, on a different lake. We agreed to take a look, and as soon as I walked into Theresa's house I knew it was the one. We quickly put an offer together, and she accepted it. She never even had to put it on the market. We sold our current home in three days to a lovely family with lots of kids.

But the story wasn't over. As beautifully as the pieces were coming together, there was one thing that had to happen first. Everything was contingent on Theresa finding a new lake house for herself. That was not going to be easy in that market.

> *God is never outdone*
> *in His generosity when you turn*
> *your thoughts over to Him.*

By now you can guess what I did. I fasted and prayed for her. Sure enough, she found the perfect home in a miraculous way, just like we had discovered ours. All three households moved two months sooner than expected, and, to this day, we remain in contact with each other. Even the realtors and bankers were a blessing to us and remain so today. Fasting brings blessing to your soul and to others. It truly is about shifting your thoughts to blessing others, which causes positive emotions that fuel the actions of praying and fasting.

God is never outdone in His generosity when you turn your thoughts over to Him. I shifted my thoughts from "not enough" to "more than enough with God," and from impossible to possible through praying and fasting for others. A community mindset of love and abundance will give you the desires of your heart.

Jesus wants to bless you, but you have to do the work of choosing better thoughts. The next time you go to Mass and tap your heart, take it seriously. Gently tap your beautiful heart and remember that it is our human fault that we are greatly sinning in our thoughts. You don't have to be sullen and guilt-ridden about this fact. God made us this way so that we would depend on Him.

> *A community mindset*
> *of love and abundance will give*
> *you the desires of your heart.*

The Penitential Act implores the help of the Virgin Mary, all the angels, and saints to pray for us to change for the good. That's eternal fire power right there. Jesus doesn't refuse His Mother. So, ask for her guidance.

The Act also implores each one of us to pray for each other to change for the good as well. Pray and bless all those around you. Start doing this at every Mass. Look around at all the other Catholics beside you in the pews. They need you. They need your good thoughts. We need each other. We are all tapping our beautiful, imperfect, stony hearts. Together we can recognize hurtful thoughts, process our emotions, and show up as our best. We are enough with God.

As the 17th century mystical poet, Thomas Traherne, writes, "To think well is to serve God in the interior court: To have a mind composed of Divine Thoughts, and set in frame, to be like Him within."[2]

VIRTUOUS ACTIONS TO CREATE GOOD HABITS

Write down one thought that might be bothering you about weight loss or fasting today. List it in the first space below. Then list the feeling that it causes in your body. What behaviors or actions do you notice when you feel that emotion? List as many as you can.

Ask yourself if this thought is helping you and blessing others. Why or why not? Re-evaluate that thought with God, asking Him how it can be shifted to help you and bless others. Write the new thought down in the space provided. Then list the new feeling that it causes in your body. What behaviors or actions do you notice when you think that thought and feel that emotion? Just becoming aware of your thoughts is the first step toward learning to process emotion and Spiritually Fast.

Current Thought:

Feeling:

Actions or Inaction:

Unwanted Result:

New Thought:

_____

_____

Feeling:

_____

_____

Actions or Inaction:

_____

_____

Result That Helps You and Blesses Others:

_____

_____

SPIRITUAL FASTING PRAYER

*Lord, I surrender my thoughts to You. I want
to love myself as You love me so that I may bless others.
I cannot do this on my own. With You, I am more than
enough. I invite You into my heart and soul. Wash me clean
of the thoughts that are not of You. Without You I can do
nothing. I know my life is not my own, it is Yours to work through
me. Lord, I am filled with gratitude for this life You've
given me. You've blessed me with enough strengths and
talents to be a Saint one day. The journey is long, but sweeter
with You and The Blessed Mother by my side. Turn my
thoughts to blessings, Oh Lord. Help me understand
how to shift all that I am into love and abundance and
bring glory to Your great name. Amen.*

CHAPTER 6

Dining In with Jesus

"He must increase, I must decrease."

—John 3:30

WOULDN'T YOU LOVE TO have dinner with Jesus?

I'm going to show you how to do this every day by asking Him into a simple intermittent fasting routine. I call it *Dining In with Jesus*. As I've explained, Spiritual Fasting is the delaying of or abstaining from food for a period of time for a spiritual purpose, and the diet world sometimes calls that practice "intermittent fasting."

This type of fasting isn't new. It has been around since before Jesus walked the earth, but our culture has taken the spiritual purpose out of it. And that's exactly why it is so difficult! I love thinking of it as *Dining in with Jesus* when I am fasting. The concept of *Dining in with Jesus* is a staple of my Delay and Pray™ method. "I'm dining in with Jesus" is a great thought that gently reminds you to keep fasting according to the food plan that you've made ahead of time.

As you probably already know, intermittent fasting involves periods of time where you are eating and drinking as usual, as well as periods of time that you are not consuming anything but water, black coffee, or tea. We call these periods eating and fasting windows.

Dining in with Jesus is another name for the fasting window or The Delay portion of the Delay and Pray™ method. It will be your fat-burning superpower if you are trying to lose weight and your energy-boosting superpower if you are looking for optimal health.

Get excited because this is the answer you've been looking for.

Intermittent fasting is challenging and requires a good mindset to achieve, but it just makes sense if you are willing to change some unwanted behaviors when it comes to overeating and overdrinking. But don't make the mistake of leaving Jesus out of the process. If some demons can only be cast out by prayer and fasting (Matthew 17:21), then you can bet what we are about to do is going to be arduous. But, it isn't worse than working toward any significant goal, like training for a 10K or graduating from college. You can discipline yourself to increase time periods without food, delaying your intake of sugar, flour, and alcohol during the week while praying your heart out.

Many people cannot go without food for even two or three hours, not for medical reasons but because they are not employing any mindset tools, not availing themselves of prayer and sacraments, or not examining what they are consuming. In the next couple chapters we are going to study food and how to easily delay it. It is The Delay that brings the miracles to your life.

Food matters. Certain foods will inhibit you from fasting well. Those foods are often highly processed and contain sugar and flour. They keep you hungry throughout the day. Foods that contain large amounts of sugar and flour fuel overdesire, overhunger, and overeating, making it difficult to fast. But you don't have to eliminate them forever. You can just delay them until Sunday.

Dining in with Jesus is "dining in" on your own body fat for a spiritual purpose. This is a way of burning fat by not eating for an extended window of time so that your body will tap into the stores of fat that you already have. This action brings the words from John 3:30 alive: "He must increase; I must decrease." Your focus upon Jesus will increase as you are praying throughout the day, and your body will decrease as you lose weight at the same time.

I learned the concept of "dining in" from Brooke Castillo at The Life Coach School. However, I added "with Jesus" to the phrase because He is the one helping us intermittently fast. Remember, we are never on our own. The Holy Spirit dwells within us from Baptism. We always can implore spiritual help in all matters, especially fasting.

My clients are seeing tremendous results in their weight loss and closeness to Christ just by delaying sugar, flour, and alcohol during the week and praying for others in the process. At first, it is challenging to delay sugar and flour from your diet because you experience physical hunger as your body transitions from sugar burning to fat burning. Your body strives to be efficient, and it will try to keep doing what it has always done. Therefore, it will take effort to switch to a different fuel source: your own fat instead of a constant intake of sugary food.

It is true that when we eat more food than we need, we gain weight. But the answer is not calorie restriction according to the old diet mentality. It is intermittent fasting. Most of us have already experienced fasting by not eating from approximately 8 pm to 8 am. This 12-hour fast happens while we are sleeping. Traditionally, we wake up, get ready for the day, and break the fast with the first meal of the day. Now it's obvious why we call this meal *break-fast*, isn't it?

The first step in mastering The Delay is to refine breakfast a bit and learn how to slowly lengthen the fasting window for a spiritual purpose. Eventually, we will be able to eat less and higher quality food between fasting windows. The healthy state I am describing here is called metabolic flexibility. That is our aim.

Metabolic flexibility is when we fat-burn most of the week and sugar-burn a little on the weekends. In this state, we can lose or maintain weight, balance hormones, lower our appetites, keep our metabolic rate speeding along, and retain our invaluable muscle mass. Fasting will help our bodies switch from one fuel source to the other with ease. The fat storage hormone called insulin facilitates this process.

> *Metabolic flexibility is when we fat-burn most of the week and sugar-burn a little on the weekends.*

I have learned to shake hands and be friends with insulin because it is so important. In other words, I understand and appreciate it. Instead of thinking about how many calories are involved in a particular food, I think in terms of my insulin levels and how it will affect my Spiritual Fasting. I want to work with my insulin levels and help my pancreas perform optimally whenever I can.

Here is a basic explanation of how insulin functions.

When we consume food, our pancreas releases insulin to deal with the rise of glucose in our bloodstream. Insulin is a fat storage hormone that directs glucose from our bloodstream into our cells, where it can be used immediately or stored in the liver and muscles as glycogen. When the liver and muscle stores become full, then the excess glucose is converted and stored as fat on our bodies to be used as energy later.

Following so far?

As the glucose levels in our bloodstream decrease over the next few hours of not eating, the pancreas releases another hormone called glucagon. This hormone signals to your liver to release glycogen from storage to maintain optimal blood glucose levels. Eventually, the glycogen in your liver and muscles becomes depleted, and that's when the fat from your fat cells converts into ketones to be used as fuel.

I feel very clear minded and energetic when I am converting fat to ketones to burn as fuel. It's the source of fuel my brain loves. When this is happening. I am in a very healthy state of ketosis. It feels so good.

Okay, here's the cheatsheet to summarize the process:

1. We eat.

2. Our bloodstream floods with glucose.

3. The pancreas releases insulin to use some glucose for immediate energy and store the leftovers as glycogen or fat for later use.

4. Then we stop eating for a while, and our bodies release glucagon.

5. The glucagon helps us use stored energy for fuel, and we operate as one healthy little human as God designed.

But, there's a problem. Most people don't stop eating or drinking. Ever.

Before researching how to Spiritually Fast using the Delay and Pray ™ method, I was always thinking about calories. I couldn't shake off the old diet mentality of calories in, calories out. So I would be drinking a skinny latte or diet cola, chewing sugar-free gum, sucking on sugar-free mints, and eating low-calorie snacks, regardless of my eating or fasting windows.

Back then, I wondered why losing weight was so difficult. I wasn't thinking in terms of insulin. Somewhere along the diet path I had started to believe that these things were free to eat any time I wanted. All these "fat-free," "sugar-free," and "calorie-free" items are not free no matter what diet you are on.

Then I swung from the "fat-free" craze in the eighties and nineties to the "full-fat" craze in the last twenty years, resulting in yo-yo dieting, bad moods, health problems, and more. I never enjoyed permanent weight loss, and I constantly struggled with Spiritual Fasting. What I didn't realize back then is that these kinds of foods elicit an insulin response when being consumed, so that the glycogen in my liver and muscles is never really depleted.

I was never entering a state of ketosis because insulin was constantly cleaning up the glucose in my bloodstream. I don't even want to mention the increased inflammation, heartburn, cholesterol, headaches, and joint pain I was causing in my body from all the sugar-free and processed food chemicals that I was consuming. An increased insulin response is causing many of the diseases that are rampant in today's society: type 2 diabetes, heart disease, and more.

If we concentrate on optimal health and permanent weight loss through Spiritual Fasting then we can stop being hungry all the time, stop working against fat burning, and stop inhibiting our ability to "keep the fast." But if we continue over-feeding ourselves into a constant state of insulin release, then we might as well just call up Jesus and let Him know that we won't be "dining in" with Him today because we have made other plans with a donut!

But there's good news. Being metabolically flexible means you don't have to give up desserts forever. Just delay them most of the time and plan them into your weekend menus.

God designed our bodies to fast. So, let's do it. Spiritual Fasting helps your body and soul work together naturally to slim down, feel better, and acquire the miracles that you've been longing for. It is time to change your focus from calories to insulin. This will help you "keep the fast" and *Dine In with Jesus* whenever you want to.[1]

One word of caution: I must note here that you should always be working with a doctor when trying out any type of fasting for the first time. If you are obese or severely overweight, you may have a higher insulin response to food than others. This is something that could hamper your fasting efforts so talk with your doctor about food intake, medications that could be working against you, possible insulin resistance, or any other medical issue. Also, if you have a history of dieting like I do, it will take you a while to feel comfortable fasting.

We will discuss the eating window in the next chapter. Remember, this isn't about restriction, it is about abundance. You can feel a little hunger and feel healthier at the same time. It just depends on the food you are consuming, whether you are eating deliberate meals instead of snacking, and if you stop eating for extended time between meals. These pieces fit together.

Think of it like this: what you eat during your eating window will help you delay food for the sake of prayer for others during your fasting window. Remember, we aren't just intermittent fasting for our own health. We are fasting for miracles, using intermittent fasting as it was originally intended—as a tool for courageous Christians. Our goal is to be healthy *and* holy. To be saints.

This new way of eating will take about two to four weeks to adopt. You may experience a withdrawal from the addiction to sugar, flour, and alcohol that your body is used to consuming. Your pallet and your brain will need time to change. Your goal is fat burning and true health, with a side of weight loss. But, after those first few weeks, you will be well on your way.

> *Our goal is to*
> *be healthy* and *holy.*

To *Dine In with Jesus* successfully, focus your thoughts on something other than food. I get out of the kitchen. One regimen I started was to schedule my sacraments at the times that I know I'll be tempted to eat. For example, I found a 5:30 pm Mass at a Church nearby. The late afternoon hours and dinner hours are my most challenging time to either keep the fast or break the fast without overeating. So now I make dinner ahead (usually after lunch when I am full), go to Mass at 5:30 pm, and come home to join my husband for dinner. Or I eat dinner beforehand (keeping the Church-prescribed one hour fast before Mass) and come home to join him while he eats dinner. The point is, I get out of the kitchen during those vulnerable moments and plan, plan, plan what I will do when I go back in. I did this when my children were little, and I even do it now when I am on vacation. No excuses.

One more thing. There is an added benefit of Spiritual Fasting that may surprise you. You will be amazed at how much you can do both spiritually and physically when you begin to *Dine In with Jesus* regularly.

There just seems to be more time.

My clients tell me they are reading more spiritual books, adding more Rosaries to their routine, and spending more time with family and friends. They are going to more Church activities, retreats, and connecting with other Christians in the community. They are learning new skills and enjoying new hobbies. They are experiencing deeper relationships and human connection rather than overeating and overdrinking, especially in the evenings. And, the best part? They are doing all of this while praying for others.

Paying attention to eating and fasting windows during your day is the key to "keeping the fast." I am always asking myself: *How do I keep* Dining In with Jesus *in the schedule I have planned so that I am able to show up in prayer and fasting for others?*

In the past, the omission of my spiritual life from my weight loss efforts was the reason why diets didn't work for me. I wasn't dieting-for-miracles. That's not a thing. It's interesting to think that I used to invite God into every area of my life except the one where I focused so much of my attention. I am so glad the Lord led me to this mission of Spiritual Fasting. It has helped me in so many ways. God increased, and I decreased. I started feeling better right away. I even started to rest more—especially on Sundays. And that is what God wanted for me all along.

I cannot stress enough that Spiritual Fasting begins by becoming aware of your thoughts. If you have been dieting for a long time, there will be subconscious thoughts and associations about fasting, as well as "good" and "bad" foods, and when and how much you can eat them. It is time to pray for wisdom, performing the Great Experiment with fasting windows and foods that are best for your body.

You may have to eliminate specific foods for a time if you find that you can't stop eating them. That's okay. You can kick out those foods from your pantry for a while, especially if you just can't resist them due to the pleasure they give you. I call these foods "runaway foods." Runaway foods are the foods that you have always reached for to comfort you and make you feel better. But what they really do is sabotage The Delay and keep you from fasting. You will be able to bring those foods back into the house later if you want, but for now get them out so you can begin this process well.

For me, runaway foods were wine, butter, crackers, peanut butter, all white flour breads and buns, cottage cheese, pretzels, Diet Coke, M&M's, chocolate chips, tortilla chips, lunchmeat, cheese slices, and white tortillas. Yep, this is my list. Your list may be different from mine. For example, someone could leave gummy bears, snickerdoodles, brownies, potato chips, and soda on my counter for days, and I wouldn't touch any of it, but they may be problematic for you. I don't negotiate with those particular foods just like I don't negotiate with cigarettes because I don't smoke. If you find yourself negotiating with runaway foods, take a break from them so you can spend your time negotiating in better ways, like when to begin and end your fasting windows. Take your struggle with runaway foods to prayer, and better yet, to adoration. Jesus will help you there.

May I suggest that unless you are buying vegetables, chicken, fish, and meat, stop buying runaway foods in bulk with the thought of saving money. You will just overeat that food item because you have so much in your cabinet. As you will learn through practice, *Dining In with Jesus* takes fortitude (courage to endure the discomfort) and lots of prudence (good decision-making). You will make it harder on yourself if you have huge bags of sugary, floury items in your cabinet and a box of wine in your fridge.

Get them out of the house. And, don't worry about your family. They will be fine. There is not a human on the planet who needs to consume candy, donuts, or chips every day. There's lots of healthy ways to get your sweet fix during the week while delaying these things to the weekend.

Okay, you get it. You can totally do this.

God created you in His image. There is only one you—your gifts, your genetics, your personality, all that you've experienced in your life up until this point. Start to love all of who you are right now. Your body is unique. This is an incredible process that will take some experimentation on your part. You will fail and try again until you figure it out.

But, you *will* figure it out.

VIRTUOUS ACTIONS TO CREATE GOOD HABITS

1. Consult the Fasting Window chart and decide on an optimal time to eat and fast.
2. Consider how you want to fold God and prayer into your daily habits.
3. Try *Dining In with Jesus*. Reflect in your journal about your experience.

SPIRITUAL FASTING PRAYER

*May our hearts crave the Living Word
and have the courage to turn toward His craving
instead of ours. We've tasted the sweetness of His love;
it really is the peace that is beyond all understanding.[2]
Worldly pleasure will ruin us if we don't let Jesus
tame our wild hearts.*

"Dining in with Jesus" Fasting Chart

Eating and Fasting Daily Chart	
Fasting Window	**Eating Window**
12	12
13	11
14	10
15	9
16	8
17	7
18	6
19	5
20	4
21	3
22	2
23	1

Shortly before joining The Delay and Pray ™ Group Coaching Experience, Jenay was the heaviest she'd ever been, and she was struggling a lot with her mental health. She had just been diagnosed with an autoimmune disorder and was struggling to manage the new difficulties in her life. She wanted to make changes in her health, but she didn't know which direction to go. She was scared because some previous weight-loss programs had done more harm than good, regarding her mindset.

Then some friends shared about Beth's powerful coaching style. They told Jenay, "Run don't walk! Go enroll in The Delay and Pray™ Group Coaching Experience! It will change your life!"

Jenay knew that Delay and Pray™ could help her turn the tide. She started working with Beth by learning the core program. Between October and February—even amidst the holiday season—she lost about 30-35 pounds.

Then she continued with the optional membership, and to date, she has lost 60 pounds. But the best part is that her body became healthy enough to try to conceive a child again.

Before Jenay found Delay and Pray ™, she regularly turned to food for comfort. She was hesitant to take her source of comfort away as she continued to deal with challenges in that season of her life. But now she looks back and sees that God was faithful to her, allowing her to experience those struggles precisely so that she could find a better way. What changed for her was the realization that her suffering could be something that was helpful to others. She could learn to take the little sufferings of denying herself sugar, flour, or alcohol, and turn them around to pray for someone in her life who was hurting.

After some time, she was surprised by how easy it was to delay—it gave her permission to desire something without giving into the desire or dealing with all the issues that come with the erroneous thought: "I can never have that food again."

Appreciation for good food is definitely a hallmark of the culture in Louisiana, where she lives. Through Delay and Pray™ she's changed her mindset completely.

"Food is language here," she reflects, "It's how we show our love. We were traveling somewhere recently, and people were like, 'You have to try the donuts at this place! They're the best donuts you'll ever eat!' and I thought, *This is so weird! Why do people talk this way about food? It's just food.*"

Jenay has found freedom in detaching from food and attaching herself to Christ in her mission. She explains that Spiritual Fasting breeds so much virtue and perseverance. This bled into every other area of her life, where she was able to detach from other idols and practice virtue beyond Spiritual Fasting.

Jenay's *Why That Makes You Cry* has been an integral part of her transformation. She continues to offer up her sacrifices and sufferings for her husband, her marriage, her kids, their future vocations, and their future spouses. Focusing on others has helped to take her out of herself and lean on God,

His mercy, and the gift of prayer. This practice of generosity and charity within her moments of suffering has been the biggest blessing of all.

CHAPTER 7

Lots of Sugar and a Little Fiber

"Do you not know that your body is the temple of the Holy Spirit within you, whom you have received from God, and that you are not your own? You have been purchased at a price. Therefore, glorify God in your body."

—1 Corinthians 6:19-20

NOW THAT WE'VE FIGURED out how to divide our day into fasting and eating windows, let's focus on the eating window.

Look around. It is obvious that we love to eat. We eat, we pray, and we love a lot. It's only a problem because overeating and overdrinking are stopping us from fasting, the cure for what ails us both physically and spiritually. Not only as individuals, but us as the Body of Christ.

If we are going to talk about what we eat, we have to start with sugar.

Not to be the bearer of bad news, but obesity is labeled as a national epidemic in the United States today.[1] More than one-third of all American adults are obese, and another third are overweight.[2] As a former math teacher, it isn't hard to calculate that this number represents most of the country.

Two-thirds.

> *Sugar will never satisfy.*
> *But abundant life will.*

And, the likely reason? Sugar. Lots of it. We are trading the sweetness of heaven for sugar. God is ready to give us so much more if we will just put down the milkshakes and pound cakes in our hands. It reminds me of Isaiah 55:2-3, in which God makes us this glorious offer: "Why spend money for that which is not bread, your wages for that which fails to satisfy. Listen carefully to me, and you will eat well and delight in rich food. Come to me and pay close attention; listen so that you may have life."

Sugar will never satisfy. But abundant life will.

Our sweet addiction came to the forefront when I began my research to figure out how to successfully Spiritually Fast. I was so surprised to read all the statistics about food-related diseases and how processed foods, filled with hidden sugar, were causing the sickness. If we want to be truly healthy, then processed food needs to be consumed in very small amounts or never again.

Therefore, in addition to the trio of sugar, flour, and alcohol, we are going to delay processed food during the week because it is a culprit in stopping us from optimal health. What is the easiest way to define processed food? It is man-made food filled with chemicals, sugar, flour, fat, and salt. It can be found in fast food restaurants or in the middle aisles of the grocery store in bags and boxes with barcodes. Processed food is tasty, intentionally manufactured to be addicting, and is marketed relentlessly because it makes so much money for manufacturers. The bottom line is, if you continue to eat processed food during your eating window, it will hinder you from *Dining In with Jesus*, Spiritual Fasting, and losing weight permanently. Again, you don't have to stop eating processed food forever. Just limit yourself to small amounts, delayed to Sundays.

Realizing the truth about hidden sugar in processed food makes me sad, as I think back to what I was feeding my little kids 20 years ago: fast food from drive-thrus, chicken nuggets, hot dogs, macaroni and cheese from a box, bread at every dinner, and dessert most nights. I cooked many homemade meals as well, but as a busy working mom, those other processed foods were weekly staples in my house.

I remember the exact year that I stopped to reconsider the food our family was eating. My oldest son started to experience migraines in high school. These headaches were debilitating and scary. My family doctor was kind and thorough but could only offer medication to remedy the situation. Trips to the emergency room were not a permanent solution, so my sister pointed me toward a functional medicine doctor and naturopathic care. After thousands of dollars of testing and amazing care not covered by insurance, he was migraine free in less than one year. We changed his diet, cleaned up his gut biome, and saw an excellent chiropractic neurologist who diagnoses and treats migraine problems and a range of disorders affecting the nervous system.

That happened over fifteen years ago and started my journey to better eating with whole foods. I started checking labels, stopped cooking casseroles with canned soups, and started serving lettuce salads loaded with fibrous vegetables. I turned desserts from sugary delights to fruit-based treats. This was a slow trajectory. At first, there was a little rebellion around the family table, but I knew it would be worth it. I was transforming myself and my loved ones from a diet mentality to a health mentality, and the lives of my children depended on it.

A few years after changing our eating, I started learning about the negative effects of sugar—not only its involvement with weight gain, but on the central nervous system and gut biome. We consume lots of sugar and a little fiber. This is killing us. All we have to do to turn our lives around is turn that sentence around: We consume lots of fiber and a little sugar.

My dream is to see this change in the next generation.

> *Your body is the temple of the Holy Spirit. We should care about what's happening in His dwelling place.*

In the last chapter we discussed reaching fat adaption through intermittent fasting. "Keeping the fast" during your fasting window is half of the equation. Healthy food consumption during your eating window is the other half, and it is just as important to your well-being. Nutrient-rich foods will keep you from becoming famished during the fasting window. So, let's get into the nitty-gritty biology of the body-soul composite and why food choices matter, especially when it comes to sugar and white flour.

Foods are made of complex compounds that affect our minds and our bodies. Every bite of food you eat does something to both aspects of you. Food affects how you feel, how well or sick you are, your mood, and your ability to move. Good food can heal your gut, reduce inflammation, enhance immune function, balance hormones, boost your detoxification system, and strengthen your bones and muscles. This is why paying attention to what you eat and drink is so important for Spiritual Fasting.

Your body is the temple of the Holy Spirit. We should care about what's happening in His dwelling place. Do you know what really happens to your food after you swallow? Let's follow a meal through the eating process beginning with our digestion so I can show you how this works.

Chewing food is the first essential step in the digestion process. Think of chewing as mechanical digestion that is performed by your teeth to help in the physical breakdown of your food. The rest of the digestion is chemical.[3] You can actually improve your health and feel better by chewing your food really well. This means putting your fork down between bites and eating slowly. This is so hard for me. Have you tried it? It's not easy, but it is a virtuous action that leads us out of the gluttony of overconsumption.

Next, the food passes from the mouth through the esophagus to the stomach. The stomach is the storage vessel that begins the breakdown process before the food moves on to the small intestine. This is done by the presence of hydrochloric acid and digestive enzymes in the stomach that are released by the body to break down the food and toxins, and kill the bacterias.

Can you see that chewed food in smaller and slower bites, lessens the amount of acid that is necessary? The more the food is broken down by the teeth, the less it will need to be broken down by the stomach. That is the goal: to make digestion easier by allowing the stomach to create just enough acid to do the job. Raw fruits and vegetables also help because they contain lots of fiber and possess their own enzymes that help to break down the food without extra work from the digestive system. Dr. Robert Lustig, author of *Fat Chance*, says this about fiber:

> "There are two types of fiber: soluble and insoluble fiber. Soluble fiber is like the pectin which holds jam together, and insoluble fiber is like cellulose (like the stringy stuff in celery). You need both—and fruit has both. When you consume both (a piece of fruit), what happens is the insoluble fiber forms a net or lattice on the inside of your intestine. Then the soluble fiber plugs the holes in the net."[4]

Dr. Lustig encourages the increase of raw fruits and vegetables for their effect on this stage of digestion. A whitish gel is formed to coat the inside of your intestine and act as a barrier so that you don't absorb all of the sugar quickly, slowing the amount of glucose entering into your bloodstream. There is sugar in the form of glucose and fructose in fruits and some vegetables, too. But, these foods are complex carbs, packed with fiber. The fiber helps slow down the absorption of glucose and fructose into the bloodstream to provide fuel for your body and for your gut biome, too.

No matter what you are eating, while it is in the stomach, food is mixed with acid until it is acidic enough to flow into the 20-foot small intestine. The small intestine is where protein, carbohydrates, and fats are broken down into nutrients and absorbed into the body by tiny fingerlike projections called *villi*.

On the villi are even tinier projections called *micro villi*. The villi work together to increase the surface area of the intestines so that our bodies can absorb as many nutrients as possible. Optimal health occurs when the villi are long and healthy so they can absorb all the nutrients we need to be healthy, strong, and feel good. I probably don't have to tell you that high sugar products do not have many nutrients. In fact, your small intestine can really only handle six to nine teaspoons of sugar at one time depending on if you are male or female. If you consume more than this amount, then the sugar is most likely passed into the large intestine where it may not be absorbed properly resulting in bloating or a feeling of heaviness in the gut. It can also sit in the intestines and ferment, leading to gas.

During this stage, the pancreas, liver, and gall bladder also release digestive enzymes and other substances to further break down the food mixture. It is here where the pancreatic enzymes break down protein (like meat or chicken) into amino acids, carbohydrates (like sweet potato and broccoli) into simple sugars that are mostly glucose, and fats (like olive oil) into short chain fatty acids.

Why is this so valuable to understand? Because the acidic material in the small intestines is vital for the release of pancreatic enzymes. Too much sugar over time will promote insulin resistance and cause the pancreas to work harder. Long term use of medications that block stomach acid can damage gut health and make you feel sick because these pancreatic enzymes are not released.

Pay close attention to what I am about to say: When we overeat and overdrink to numb discomfort, we reach for Alka Seltzer and other acid blockers to recover. And, those medications help in the short term, but they also create a losing cycle that keeps us stuck in the long run. The answer? By now, it should come as no surprise.

You will stop the cycle when you stop overeating and overdrinking by delaying sugar, flour, alcohol, and processed foods to Sundays in small amounts.

The last stop on the digestive journey is the large intestine. It is wider and only about five feet long. It takes what is passed from the small intestine and absorbs the water from the food mixture. Too little water absorbed leads to diarrhea, and too much leads to constipation. For the most part, the absorption of nutrients occurs in the small intestine. So, whatever is left of the chicken, sweet potato, and broccoli that can't be digested (such as fiber, waste substances, bacteria, and undigested food) are now feces that will exit your body.

Why am I sharing this? Because now you can imagine your food going through your body from mouth to toilet. Think of chicken, broccoli, and sweet potato going through the digestive system, making all the stops and transitions along the way, while releasing nutrients and creating the energy you need to be fantastic all day.

But wait. What about a donut?

As you can imagine a donut goes through the same process, but there is no nutrition to fuel your precious body. In fact, that donut is likely working against you, increasing the acid in your stomach, spiking the glucose levels in your bloodstream, increasing your insulin production, compounding your fat storage, and creating a leaky gut. On top of that, you will be hungrier and less likely to move around after eating it.[4]

Our food affects our digestion. Our digestion affects how healthy we are and also how we feel, both physically and emotionally. Think of this the next time you reach for that snack. How will it affect your gut? Is it worth it? The taste will give you great momentary pleasure, for sure. But the long term effects may not be helpful. In the Great

Experiment of Spiritual Fasting, you get to be the one to decide.

Hormones will help you make that decision.

The first hormone you can make friends with is insulin, the miracle fat-storage hormone.

As I mentioned in the previous chapter, the pancreas releases insulin to take care of the glucose in your bloodstream. Insulin is a life-saver because we cannot survive too much glucose in our blood. Simply put, insulin takes the excess glucose not needed for energy at the time and stores it away for energy later, in the form of glycogen and eventually, fat. If you don't exercise, you never need to use that extra energy, and fat just accumulates in your body.

This brings us to another friendly hormone that is ready to cooperate and bring you to optimal health: leptin. Leptin sends a signal to your brain and body that you are full and you should stop eating and go exercise or move.

Insulin and leptin are good friends;
they depend on one another.
But they also like to hang out with
one other hormone: ghrelin.

When you have too much insulin in your blood, it blocks the hormone called leptin. If leptin is not working properly, you have a tendency to overeat and then go lay on the couch. Leptin helps regulate your metabolism and the rate of fat breakdown. You want leptin working at full speed in your body. As leptin levels rise, your metabolic rate increases. As leptin levels fall, your metabolism slows. Too much sugar increases insulin therefore decreases leptin, telling your body it is starving and to eat and conserve energy.

But leptin is not just about weight loss. It is about living the full, healthy life that God intended for you. Leptin is a hormone made by fat cells in response to energy levels. It travels to various organs in the body to let them know there is enough fuel on board to engage in high-energy metabolic processes. Some of these high-energy activities include: puberty, pregnancy, and creating strong bones. If your leptin is blocked or low, all of these important functions could be limited. The whole body utilizes leptin.[5]

Insulin and leptin are good friends; they depend on one another. But they also like to hang out with one other hormone: ghrelin.

Ghrelin is your hunger hormone, the one that lets you know you are hungry. And high insulin levels increase the production of ghrelin. If this happens, then you are more apt to overeat. The more sugar, flour, alcohol, and processed food you consume, the more you want to consume. It's not your fault. The ghrelin is telling you that you are hungry.

This is the reason why many people have a difficult time with Spiritual Fasting. They can't make it through a 12-hour fasting window because they are so hungry. It isn't real hunger because they have enough glycogen and fat storage to last for days. They are hungry (and even "hangry!") because the hormone ghrelin is practically screaming inside them.

They have become sugar burners.

When the body predominantly uses sugar for energy it is called sugar-burning. The body gets in the habit of craving sugar for quick energy and never reaches into its energy storage of glycogen and fat. The opposite of sugar-burning is fat-burning, or fat-adaption, and it is our goal. Fat adaption is where we choose fat-burning during the week and delay sugar-burning to Sundays.

By delaying sugar, flour, alcohol, and processed foods, we are training our bodies to transition smoothly back and forth between fat-adaption and sugar-burning, allowing us to stay in a comfortable state called metabolic flexibility.

Metabolic flexibility takes practice to master, but taking the first step is easy. Say it with me now: Lots of fiber and a little sugar.

VIRTUOUS ACTIONS TO CREATE GOOD HABITS

A *protocol* is a set of rules and procedures. Establishing a food protocol for yourself is an important tool in Spiritually Fasting. Let's begin by considering what you typically eat and drink during the day and record all the food that you usually consume in the space provided. Note the amounts and the times that you eat it. Include meals, snacks, beverages, and water consumption.

The next day, write down how you could substitute vegetables, healthy fats and grains, and protein for any processed food or sugary items on the list. Consider what it would take for you to do this Monday through Saturday. What thoughts come up for you around delaying processed food or sugary items to Sundays every week? Examine your use of over-the-counter antacids like Tums and Alka Seltzer. Why and when are you taking these medications? What foods or beverages and what quantities are you consuming before taking them? Record this information for yourself over time. Do your own digestion research and talk with your doctor about the symptoms you are having that precipitate the need for antacids. We are a nation hooked on antacids, and we pop them often without thinking of why we are doing this and what the long term effects are.

Take time to wonder and pray with confidence that you will figure this out with God's help. God is on your side and wants the best for your precious body that He designed. He would never have created Spiritual Fasting if it wasn't optimal for both body and soul.

SPIRITUAL FASTING PRAYER

Father, thank you for having made my body in such a way as to be able to use the fruits of the earth and so develop and serve you. Thank you, Father, for all those who through their work produce new life possibilities. Thank you for those who have much and give away to others. Thank you for all who are hungry for heavenly bread while eating this earthly one. Father, thank you for all those who have nothing to eat today for I am convinced that you will send them help through good people. Amen.

—Fr. Barbaric Slavko, *Pray with the Heart!*[16]

CHAPTER 8

Feasting on Life

"For God did not give us a spirit of timidity, but rather a spirit of power and of love, and of wisdom."

—2 Timothy 1:7

DELAYING INSTEAD OF DENYING is great news. The Delay and Pray™ method of eating sugar, flour, and alcohol only on Sundays works well because we humans love patterns and operating within a regimen. For this program, I use an Eat, Fast, Feast Cycle (EFF) that I learned from *Eat Fast Feast* by Jay Richards.[1] He taught me to form a virtuous habit around a daily and weekly pattern that my body and soul could adhere to. While his program focuses on the biology of metabolic flexibility, the Delay and Pray™ method combines it with a spiritual and physical purpose.

The beauty of the feast is that it is a wonderful time to glorify God in our bodies while appreciating the bounty of the food of the earth in moderation. Virtue is best lived out in moderation in all things.

Saint Bernard's advice is a good guide for your day of feasting: "Keep to the middle if you wish to keep moderation. The midway is the safe way. Moderation abides in the mean, and moderation is virtue. Every abiding place outside the bounds of moderation is only exile to the wise man."[2]

> *The beauty of the feast*
> *is that it is a wonderful time*
> *to glorify God in our bodies*
> *while appreciating the*
> *bounty of the food of*
> *the earth in moderation.*

Here is how EFF works:

- **Eat normally on Monday, Tuesday, Thursday, and Saturday.**
  - Eating normally looks like planning your meals ahead of time, while delaying sugar, flour, processed food, and alcohol. Eat in one, two, or three meals, with no snacking. These are the days of love and abundance. You are loving yourself by consuming nourishing foods, as well as loving others with your sacrifice and prayers.

- **Fast on Wednesday and Friday because this is an ancient custom of the Church.**
  - Fasting means abstaining from meat and eating either

less food or less often (longer fasting windows of consuming only water, unsweet tea, and black coffee). These are the days of deep prayer for others.

- **Feast on Sunday and solemnities (including vigils) because these days are Feast Days and a celebration of the Eucharist and the life, death, and resurrection of Jesus Christ.**

  - Feast to celebrate the resurrection of the Lord with small amounts of sugar, flour, processed food, or alcohol beginning with Saturday night after Mass. Stop the feast when you have had enough. *Enough* begins in your body—you will start to feel a sensation when you are full enough to stop eating. Then use a sound mind to choose to stop.

As you begin the healthy rhythm of EFF, it is important to clarify that feasting is not bingeing or eating and drinking everything you want. You won't be delaying all of your desires throughout the week, just to gorge yourself on the weekends. That won't work. You will feel terrible every Monday morning.

And you will miss the point of the feast.

Think of every Sunday or solemnity as a Little Easter. There is no need for fasting or delaying as we celebrate the risen Lord! This is great news, but don't get in the drive-thru line just yet. First, let's take a closer look at feasting. Here are a few definitions of feasting that resonate with me:

- *to dwell with gratification or delight*
- *a rich or abundant meal*

- *something highly agreeable*
- *eat sumptuously (splendid, opulent, magnificent)*

Do these definitions describe your typical fast food experience? Not in my world.

I think of feasting as a juicy steak, a baked potato, a glass of wine, and one of my favorite salads, filled with cashews and croutons. When it comes to food, this type of meal brings me gratification and delight. The ingredients are splendid. I take the time to enjoy every moment, striving to eat just enough to glorify God in my celebration. This is my plan for Sundays and solemnities because it works. Sunday is the highest solemnity, and for me, the greatest feast day where I celebrate the Mass and Eucharist. Mass comes alive for me now. The experience is profound as I attend in awe of what Jesus has suffered for me and my family. After a week of delaying and praying, I come to Sunday Mass in reverence, awe, and total thanksgiving. He is the Way, the Truth, and the Life,[5] and He is our greatest Feast.

So instead of overconsuming food on feast days, slowly adopt the mindset of "feasting on life:"

- Celebrate the sacraments.
- Take in the wonderous scriptures and apply them to your life.
- Cook amazing meals that are appealing and satisfying to the tastebuds.
- Plan fun activities and savor the connection with your loved ones.
- Move your body and plan great recreational activities to enjoy the beauty of nature.
- Rest and thank God for the power of your mind and the miracle of your body.

- Lean into the wisdom of the Church.
- Go out and spread the Good News of the Gospel just like the Apostles.

My friends, feasting on life is true feasting.

One of my clients who just finished the Delay and Pray ™ Group Coaching Experience told me that a friend recently said she was glowing with a positive energy that could almost be felt. That is the power of the Holy Spirit coursing through us to serve the whole world. He wants to glow and flow through all of us. This can be done with Spiritual Fasting! Let Him flow through you, even when you feast in celebration on Sundays.

> *My friends, feasting on life is true feasting.*

If you are new to Spiritual Fasting, don't be dismayed if you overindulge at first. Your experience of feasting will be created over time. Our memories and past experiences typically associate feasts with lots of food. But it doesn't have to be all about the food.

Begin with the question: "How do I desire to celebrate the resurrected Lord?" Your personal definition of feasting on life will develop from there.

Part of my personal definition of feasting on life is growing in virtue. Through EFF, paired with life coaching, this started happening for me. I became aware of my God-given temperament, discovering my natural virtues of zeal for souls, fortitude, diligence, leadership, and enthusiasm. At the same time, I also discovered my weaknesses of control, anger, pride, and ungodly self-reliance. I wasn't great at processing my emotions or waiting. When Wednesdays and Fridays would roll around, I would get very anxious about limiting my food intake. Not drinking on Friday nights made me anxious, too. At first, all of this was extremely uncomfortable. Because I am an energetic person with passionate emotions, I would get angry about the delay and then eat or drink off protocol. You could say that I had a short fuse. I didn't think I could change that personality trait in me. I thought it was the temperament that I was stuck with, and I disliked myself a lot.

> You can always "choose your hard."

Then I realized that my temperament was a blessing and gift from God. It offered me a chance to examine myself and intentionally conform to the likeness of Christ. After praying for the virtues of patience, humility, meekness, and lots of prudence, my anxiety lessened. I started to slow down. I stopped choosing to be angry. I started choosing love. The emptier I became on fasting days, the more loving I became. The more loving I became, the easier EFF became.

Please don't refrain from trying the Delay and Pray ™ method because it is hard in the beginning. You can always "choose your hard." So do you want hard now or hard later? My advice is to choose hard now. Accept the short-term difficulty of Spiritual Fasting, and you won't regret it. The alternative is to accept the long-term difficulty that an unhealthy lifestyle brings.

Why is fasting so difficult? Because fasting from food is more demanding on you than giving time or money. You are giving your body and your flesh. It is not easy to be hungry—even just a little bit.

It takes Jesus, preparation, thought, commitment, and community to do it well.

> *Eventually, you will discover*
> *that you love life*
> *more than you love food.*

Oh, and it takes the willingness to try.

Eventually, you will discover that you love life more than you love food.

VIRTUOUS ACTIONS TO CREATE GOOD HABITS

In the space provided, reflect on the following questions:

How could you plan to eat just enough?

_____

_____

_____

_____

How could you fast?

_____

_____

_____

_____

Redefine *feasting* for yourself. What could feasting on life look like for you?

_____

_____

_____

_____

SPIRITUAL FASTING PRAYER

*Heavenly Father, as I begin this time of fasting,
I pray that You will fill me with Your grace, and grant me
strength and resolution to endure the hunger and discomforts
that I may experience during this fast.*

*Keep me strong and alert, Lord. Deliver me from
all unwanted thoughts and distractions that would
jeopardize my fast. Protect me from temptation and
from the Evil One. May this fast lead me to spiritual growth,
renewal, and healing.*

*Grant me, Father, the assurance that You will
strengthen me during the difficult and challenging times of this
fast, and meet me for sweet moments of spiritual growth and
surrender. Help me to focus not on what is being taken away, but
what I will be gaining as I use this fast as a spiritual discipline.*

With you leading me, Holy Spirit, I am ready.

*My God, I offer up this fast to You and to Your glory. May Your
mercy be always upon me, a sinner.*

In Jesus' name I pray. Amen.[4]

Stefanie was at a health crossroads in her life immediately before joining the Delay and Pray™ Group Coaching Experience. She had been working with a functional medicine nutritionist to help heal her gut from serious food poisoning five years earlier.

The nutritionist had advised her to start tracking her macros, and she absolutely hated it. It felt too much like the same diet mentality that she had encountered all her life: she was always thinking about the diet program rather than thinking about God. Eventually, it struck her how diet programs encouraged people to treat their diet like a golden calf. She didn't want to worship what she ate, and she wasn't losing any weight by tracking her macros.

While visiting her parents in Florida, she looked for an inspirational podcast to listen to while she went for a walk. She came across an episode where Beth had been interviewed, and as Stefanie listened to Beth explain the Delay and Pray ™ method, she thought to herself, "This is the coolest thing ever. This is amazing. This is exactly what I'm looking for."

Stefanie decided to join Beth's program. She didn't want to tell anybody about what she was doing, though. She had already tried so many things to lose weight over the years, and she didn't know if people would understand why she was trying one more thing. Stefanie had been really involved with her Parish and a women's Scripture study course, so she told her husband it was just a different women's group.

As she worked through the program, she was very surprised by how weight was just falling off. She wasn't counting calories. She wasn't doing any of the typical "diet things." She kept asking herself, "How is this working?" Every week, she was seeing results, and she was overjoyed.

Then the emotional storm hit.

In a short time period, her dad was diagnosed with cancer, her seven-year-old dog unexpectedly died, and her oldest child headed off to college.

Stefanie believes that if she had just been doing a typical weight-loss program with a diet mentality, she would have slipped back into her old ways, but she was able to hold onto the spiritual framework of the program and use it to help her get through that difficult period. She didn't turn to overeating. She turned to God, while praying and fasting for her dad and other loved ones. Despite the emotional storm, she still lost 15 pounds.

One of the special answers to prayers came through the woman who cleans her dad's house, who happens to be Catholic. When the woman learned he had cancer, she immediately stopped what she was doing and started praying for him on the spot. Stefanie knew the moment had been heaven-sent.

"Just prior to that, I had been praying for something special to happen to bring comfort and help to my dad because I couldn't be there with him. As soon as he told me that someone had prayed for him right there in his house, I thought, 'Oh my gosh! that's an answer to my prayer!'"

CHAPTER 9

The Vice and Virtue Cycles

"'All things are lawful for me,' but not all things are beneficial. 'All things are lawful for me,' but I will not allow myself to be dominated by anything."

—1 Corinthians 6:12

DID YOU RUN OUT of printer paper or batteries? Shop online, and the package will show up on your doorstep tomorrow. Don't feel like eating what's in your fridge? Order a meal with an app on your phone, and within the hour, a driver will bring it to you. Someone screwed up your project at work? Get angry and talk about it behind her back. Too tired to go to confession this month? Just stay home; He knows you're sorry.

All of these instant-gratification responses give us a quick reward. The more we seek short-term comfort, the more we set ourselves up for long-term pain. That is a description of a life of vice. The quick results may have seemed harmless in the beginning, but in various ways, we are repeating the same detrimental behaviors over and over again. Without realizing it, we are programming ourselves to stay in a Vice Cycle. Yet, God wants us to seek short-term discomfort to set ourselves up for long-term freedom. That is a description of a life of virtue. When we start managing our thoughts with the help of grace to change our feelings and behaviors, we enter the Virtue Cycle.

Why would we keep choosing vice over virtue? It is due, in part, to dopamine.

> *The more we seek short-term comfort, the more we set ourselves up for long-term pain.*

Dopamine is a hormone that feels good and is highly motivating. Because of our reliance on dopamine, we are forming reward pathways based on instant gratification, and they have become the dominant drivers in our lives. That is not what God intended.

Does this mean that dopamine is bad? No! Without dopamine, we would die. We need it in moderate amounts. And the more we learn about it the better. For one thing, you may find it interesting that dopamine is more about *wanting* than *getting*. Scientists say that this critical hormone is linked much closer to the anticipation of a reward than to the actualization of the reward.[1] Think back to a time when you really wanted something, but when you finally got it, it wasn't as good as you had anticipated. That's the feeling of dopamine at work in your body and brain.

When you want to consume sugar, flour, and alcohol, the

increasing desire triggers the release of dopamine. That makes you feel good and creates even more desire. Then when you satisfy that craving with eating or drinking, your brain experiences a larger dopamine hit that causes an overwhelming sensation of pleasure. Take note of the fact that only the first one or two bites are satisfying. The pleasure diminishes the more you consume the "reward" that you had wanted so badly only a moment before. As a result, you will start feeling an "overdesire" for these foods as you chase false satisfaction.

What is happening here?

Simply put, we are addicted to dopamine. Dr. Anna Lembke, author of *Dopamine Nation*, describes how we are bombarded by instant-gratification opportunities that keep us in a state of constant pleasure-seeking. This constant high dopamine state will eventually cause great pain as we experience anxiety, restlessness, exhaustion, and stress from stopping the behavior. As soon as the "dopamine drip" ceases, we feel discomfort, even suffering.

High dopamine triggers are easy to get and result in high highs and low lows. Some examples of high dopamine triggers are: sugar, flour, alcohol, processed food, overeating, overdrinking, screens, cell phone use, isolation, inactivity, lying, gossiping, self-reliance, faithlessness, overwhelm, and indecision.

Low dopamine triggers result in steady highs and steady lows. Some examples of low dopamine triggers are: whole food, exercise, sacraments, prayer, delaying, nature, connection, friendship, telling the truth, managing thoughts and emotions, fat adaptation, and fasting.

I call the high dopamine triggers *cheap dopamine* and the low dopamine triggers *expensive dopamine*. The concept of cheap and expensive dopamine has solved so many problems for me. It explains why sugar, flour, processed foods, and alcohol are so hard to delay. For some of us, these foods foster an addiction and solidify a reward pathway that creates cravings all week long.

> *I call the high dopamine triggers* cheap dopamine *and the low dopamine triggers* expensive dopamine.

Addiction is defined as the continued compulsive use of the substance or behavior, regardless of harm to self or others.[2] So let's be clear, I am not clinically addicted to any of the substances mentioned above, but they can be idols in my life. If I'm honest, each one is a "golden calf" that I prefer over reaching out to God. Why? Because, in my fallen mind, He is taking too long with ... whatever I am waiting for. I'd rather not be patient and suffer well. So I go for the cheap dopamine so I can get a big bang for little effort. If I do not work on interrupting that reward pathway then my weight will go up and down like an elevator. I will be overdesiring food all week, while being less yoked with Jesus.

Thank God for Spiritual Fasting. Because I focused on mastering the principles of the Delay and Pray™ method, I went from the Vice Cycle to the Virtue Cycle over time. I could never have transformed myself. Jesus, through His grace, takes me there daily. At the end of this chapter, you will find a simple diagram to help you understand how the Vice and Virtue Cycles work.

Let's start with The Vice Cycle of Daily Sugar, Flour, and Alcohol. This pattern is fueled by cheap dopamine. It is a vicious cycle, making it difficult to eat whole food with a spiritual purpose, Spiritually Fast, and be compassionate with yourself and others. There is plenty of judgment, comparison and despair in the mix because The Vice Cycle always revolves around "me."

The Vice Cycle begins when the daily consumption of sugar, flour, processed food, and alcohol results in overdesire. You want a quick fix, and you want it now! As we have discussed in a previous chapter, that is because the large amounts of glucose in your bloodstream releases insulin, which tells ghrelin (The "I'm Hungry" Hormone) to get loud and tells leptin (The "I'm Full" Hormone) to stay quiet. Ghrelin transfers the desire in your brain to physical "overhunger," and your stomach has pangs or growls ... even though you ate recently. Have you ever wondered why that was happening? It is due to overhunger. Those pangs feel very real, but logically, you know it doesn't make sense. The overhunger is so strong that the only realistic response is overeating. Instead of a handful of chips, you eat the whole bag. Instead of one cookie, you eat four. Instead of a scoop of ice cream, you eat the entire pint, straight from the container. Notice that all of these foods are processed, chock full of sugar and flour. You know what that means. Consuming all of that sugar, flour, and alcohol will repeat the circuit, and soon enough, the overdesire will kick in again. I call this The Vice Cycle because it is the breeding ground of sloth and gluttony.

On the other hand, The Virtue Cycle is available to you. It is fueled by expensive dopamine. It is a good cycle that always has a spiritual purpose involved, making it easy to be oriented toward compassion with yourself and others. There is plenty of wonder, curiosity, and confidence in God's ability to help. Coaching, grace, and awareness of your thoughts help you stay in this cycle.

The Virtue Cycle begins when delaying sugar, flour, processed food, and alcohol results in True Desire, which is the love of Jesus and others. True Desire is the opposite of overdesire. You want the answer to your prayers more than anything else. And as you pray from a place of True Desire, ordered eating becomes your normal way of approaching food. The less glucose in your bloodstream, the less insulin floods your body. Ghrelin tells you that you are hungry only when it is true, and after you have eaten some nutritious food, leptin tells you that you are full. Before you realize it, you are eating to "enough." You no longer clean your plate for the sake of it. You notice the signals your body is sending. This helps you to delay sugar, flour, and alcohol consistently, which keeps you in a pattern that benefits you in the end. I call it The Virtue Cycle because it develops the virtues of diligence and temperance.

> *God designed our bodies to balance. He is a God of Order. Virtue is the heavenly homeostasis that we are looking for.*

Here's another way to look at how dopamine affects your behaviors, as summarized from *Dopamine Nation*. Think of a scale with pain on one side and pleasure on the other. If I eat a chocolate chip cookie, I get a release of dopamine in my reward circuitry. My brain balance tips to the side of pleasure. The brain then regulates the dopamine to push the pleasure side of the scale back up, and that means the other side experiences pain for a while. I have two options— eat another cookie to send myself back into pleasure or stop eating, pray, and let the discomfort pass. If I choose the latter, eventually the scale will balance by itself.

With this analogy in mind, you can imagine that if I eat ten or twenty cookies, bringing extreme pleasure, I will have to endure the same amount of pain and discomfort to level back up to balance. This period of discomfort can be described as the hangover, the after effect, and the desire for "seconds." It's overeating and overdrinking even though you know you have had enough. If you train yourself to not consume more immediately and just delay and pray through the regulation (I call it a dopamine dip) for seconds or minutes or hours, the feeling of craving will pass.

But, you have to wait for balance.

God designed our bodies to balance. He is a God of Order. Virtue is the heavenly homeostasis that we are looking for—moderate pleasure balanced by moderate discomfort. Unfortunately, as we have grown away from God and the study of virtue, we have forgotten obedience and the concept of moderation. We don't attend the sacraments as often as we need to fill up our souls with grace and are left with neural pathways that demand instant gratification and pleasure at a large cost to our body-soul composite. We are out of balance—tipped toward pleasure, resulting in constant pain in its various forms.

We have traded virtue for vice. We're losing diligence and gaining sloth, accepting gluttony and discarding temperance. No wonder poor mental and physical health have become epidemic.

The good news is that we can turn around overdesire, overhunger, and overeating through delaying and praying.

Slowly but surely we can balance the scale.

VIRTUOUS ACTIONS TO CREATE GOOD HABITS

Look closely at the following illustrations of The Vice and Virtue Cycles. In the space provided, reflect on the ways that The Vice Cycle and The Virtue Cycle show up in your life.

_____

_____

_____

_____

_____

_____

_____

_____

_____

_____

_____

_____

_____

SPIRITUAL FASTING PRAYER

Lord, I need Your help in turning my heart to You in discomfort instead of reaching for food and alcohol that I can delay. I want to be hungry for You and make space for Your divine presence so that I may fulfill the mission that You have for me on this earth. My body is precious to You. My heart longs for You. Heal my addictions so that I may live a long and healthy life dedicated to virtue and moderation. Help me find a community that will help me heal and stop the temptation toward overdesire. Lead me to the sacraments and prayer where I can dwell with You in your glory and be made the temple of your grace once and for all.

The Vice Cycle of Daily SFA*- Keeps us from God

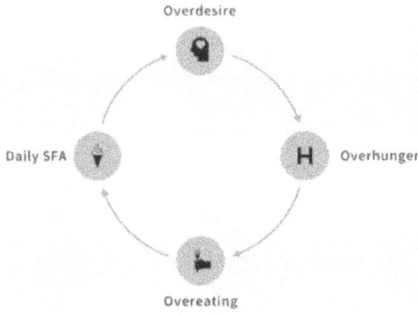

- SFA ⬆ Glucose Insulin Ghrelin ⬆
- Insulin ⬆ Leptin ⬇
- Sloth - *Laziness* ⬆
- Gluttony - *Overconsumption* ⬆

Overdesire

Daily SFA

Overhunger

Overeating

The Virtue Cycle of Spiritual Fasting - Draws us towards God

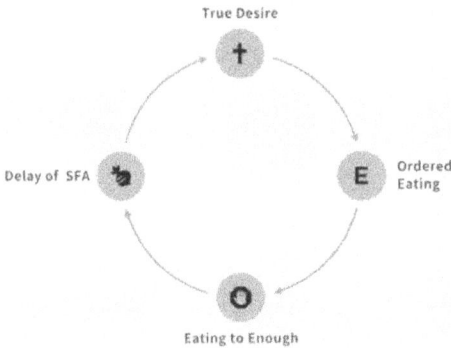

- SFA ⬇ Glucose Insulin Ghrelin ⬇
- Insulin ⬇ Leptin ⬆
- Diligence ⬆
- Temperance ⬆

True Desire

Delay of SFA

Ordered Eating

Eating to Enough

* Sugar, Flour, Alcohol

CHAPTER 10

The Answer Is in the Church

"Prayer knocks at the door, fasting obtains,
and mercy receives."

—St. Chrysologus[1]

I WENT THROUGH A period of loneliness when I started my coaching business. I put in long hours developing and writing my course, setting up the business, establishing the website and IT functions, hiring staff, and so much more. My business is also my mission so I was glad to throw everything I had into it. Until one day, after working tirelessly for two years, I looked up from my computer and realized that I was unsatisfied. Sure, I was getting physically and spiritually fit, and I was on my way to reaching my financial goals, but I was really unhappy.

Because I was lonely.

Most of my life was online. My coaching was online. My writing was online. Honestly, everything was online. I was working from sunup to sundown, and isolated while doing so.

Oddly enough, those isolated patterns can be addicting. I was getting comfortable with the pain. I was still spending time with my husband and connecting with my children often, but when it came to my career, I felt like I was on the computer all the time! It was easier to work alone rather than slow down to include others because, hey, I had goals to fulfill. At least, that was what I kept telling myself. Every once in a while, I would throw in a "This is all for Jesus," for good measure. Of course, it was. But there was never an end to the to-do list. And I could get so much more done without a commute or changing out of my leggings. Everything was very efficient when I worked from home.

Then, the isolation I had tolerated in my professional life began to seep into my personal life. I was no longer seeking out community and friendships within the Church. As I look back, the active life that I lived before the Covid fiasco had slowly melted away. I would even get frustrated with daily Mass if it went too long, or if the priest decided to sing an extra stanza at the beginning.

I'd be thinking, *Come on! Let's get going, Father. I have to get back home!*

In this book, you have discovered how certain foods can be addictive. Be aware that work and isolation can be mildly addictive, too. We can attach ourselves to our comfort zones, thinking that they bring us joy. Maybe that reminds you of a Christmas song, but "tidings of comfort and joy" come from Christ alone, not from what we think we need. We have started to confuse all kinds of selfish things for comfort and joy ... and then we wonder why we feel so lonely.

It's counterfeit comfort and phony joy.

Our nationwide addiction to isolated work brings a low level of chronic sadness. Have you felt it? When it started bothering me deeply, I found myself in adoration week after week, praying for some sanity and a solution. In my mind, I thought I had to work many focused hours to get my business running. I had almost become prideful at the amount of effort I was putting in and the Spiritual Fasting I could achieve.

> *Our nationwide addiction*
> *to isolated work brings a*
> *low level of chronic sadness.*

Then Jesus reminded me that something was missing. Once again, He was calling me out of self-reliance and into surrender. He was calling me out of my home and into the Church. He was calling me away from my screens and into fellowship.

It was a lesson I had learned before.

Three years prior, my mom had just died. I felt torn apart. During Lent that year, I had decided to eliminate all sugar, flour, processed food, and alcohol from my diet, go to Mass as often as I could, attend every Lenten talk I could find in the evenings, and pray my heart out. I was compelled to go deep within and walk the road of Calvary in my grief. I snugged under the cross with Jesus, uniting my daily cross with His. There I would plead for healing, forgiveness, and for the restoration of relationships. I knew only Jesus could do this impossible task.

One evening I was alone in the Church waiting for the speaker. While reading a beautiful spiritual book, I started to cry. I could feel the healing presence of the Lord. I looked up at the crucifix and heard Jesus whisper in my heart, "Rest in the wound in My side."

He wanted me to surrender.

> *Just like God brought Eve*
> *from Adam's side, He brought*
> *the Church from Jesus's side.*

I had never contemplated the Lord's side wound before. But when the speaker began his talk a few minutes later, wouldn't you know he discussed that very thing? He quoted one of the Doctors of the Church, Oregen: "Christ has flooded the universe with divine and sanctifying waves. For the thirsty he sends a spring of living water from the wound which the spear opened in His Side. From the wound in Christ's side has come forth the Church, and He has made her His Bride."[2]

Just like God brought Eve from Adam's side, He brought the Church from Jesus's side.

It was obvious. The Lord was telling me to always take safe refuge in the side wound of the Catholic Church, where I would find all the answers to my problems. He was asking me to come back daily and build community. It was at that very moment that I realized fellowship is always available. Eventually, I would even see my Mom again, but she was with me in spirit, even now.

The Church is the place where we can seek the hidden Jesus in all the sacraments, where the last joyful mystery of finding the Child Jesus in the temple is played out in our very lives.

That revelation changed me.

So when I was struggling with loneliness and overwork in my business, the Lord brought His side wound to my mind once again. It was time to apply Truth and get into fellowship with others. I understand that screens and some isolation will always be a part of my coaching business, but I make the effort to put the business in God's hands and work my hours intentionally, as I rekindle old friendships and invest in new ones.

When I am participating in the sacramental life of the Church and living in community with others, I feel better, and I don't have to turn to food for comfort and joy.

The result is that my happiness has returned, and the business has doubled in success. Now I am back to flooding my life with friends and family. Some of these amazing humans I've known all my life, but others are friends I've recently met. My husband and I have immersed ourselves into an active group of Catholic people. We are playing golf, pickleball, boating, attending weekly scripture study, enjoying family gatherings, networking at Catholic business events, and seeking out more charitable activities.

When I am participating in the sacramental life of the Church and living in community with others, I feel better, and I don't have to turn to food for comfort and joy. God has made us for Himself. We are created to be in community with Him and His image-bearers. We want to feed our souls with grace from the sacraments and come face-to-face with each other within the Body of Christ.

We need *both* aspects of the Church because we are body and soul.

Our Catechism states: "The human body shares in the dignity of 'the image of God:' it is a human body precisely because it is animated by a spiritual soul, and it is the whole human person that is intended to become, in the body of Christ, a temple of the Spirit" (CCC 364).

Our bodies and souls are integrated and united as our whole being, not to be separated until earthly death. We are the temple of the Holy Spirit. As we care deeply for our bodies, we must also care for our souls. Our souls mysteriously contain our minds so it is worth trying to understand our minds. Why? Because, as we know, our thoughts affect our results! And that doesn't apply only to our thoughts about food. Let's take a closer look at your thoughts about the Church:

Are you always thinking you'll start going back to Church next week?

Do you worry that it is too hard to make new friends at Church?

Are you sick of the same people in the same groups at Church?

Do you think Church activities are boring?

Do you think some people in Church leadership are weird?

Are you treating Church like a drive-thru because there is no real friendship there for you?

Do you constantly tell yourself that you are too busy to get involved in the Church?

These thoughts may seem innocent, and some may even be true, but they are not helping you. So let's shine some light on your mind to see what's happening here. In Ephesians 5:13-14, we read that "everything that is exposed by the light is made visible, and whatever is made visible is light. Therefore, it is said,

'Awake, O sleeper!
Rise from the dead,
and Christ will shine on you.'"

If we want to live an abundant life, it's time to wake up and shine a light on what is actually happening in this complicated mind of ours!

St. Thomas Aquinas explains the mind better than anyone. But you may not have time to read his lengthy treatise on the Ontological Man so here is a quick summary of his work.

He asserts that our mind is composed of three parts. We possess a lower intellect called the Passive Intellect, a higher intellect called the Possible Intellect, and the Agent Intellect functions as a messenger in-between the two.

The Passive Intellect is in the material part of the brain that is your body. It comprises the common sense powers which are your five senses: sight, hearing, smell, taste, and touch. Within this material part of the brain also resides the imagination, memory, associations, and appetites, which are our emotions. The Passive Intellect draws in outside experiences from your common sense powers and consolidates them, sending them to three places:

Imagination that draws on past and present images.

Memory that combines past and present memories.

Cogitative power that draws on past and present associations.

This Passive Intellect is called the battlefield of the mind because the demons can actually access the material part of the mind. They can nudge our imaginations and lower faculties. Why does this happen? Because at the Fall of Man, Adam and Eve conceded this material part of our intellect over to Satan through their disobedience to God. But all is not lost. Through baptism by grace, in the name of Jesus, we can reclaim the territory of our minds and take back the terrain to become saints.

What great news! If the enemy can move our imaginations toward the negative, the Holy Spirit can move them toward the positive. Invoke the spiritual realm into your thoughts for help every day. This explains why we ask or plead for the intercession of the Most Holy Blessed Mother, the holy angels and saints, Saint Michael the Archangel, and Saint Joseph, who is the terror of Demons. Their intercession really does help you.

As you can see, there's a lot more going on in the Passive Intellect than you may have realized.

> *If the enemy can move*
> *our imaginations toward the*
> *negative, the Holy Spirit can move*
> *them toward the positive.*

The Agent Intellect comes into play when it passes a thought from the Passive Intellect to the Possible Intellect.

The Possible Intellect is in the immaterial part of the brain that is your soul. It is the higher function of our minds, where we think about our thinking. This is where our thoughts can be tested. Humans are the only beings with this capability. Animals do not have the power to examine their thoughts. Only image-bearers of God can stop and look at the thoughts that are racing around in our Passive Intellect to judge and decide whether they are ultimately for our highest good. The Possible Intellect stops to ask why. *Why am I thinking that thought? Why am I doing what I am doing? Is this thought true and good?* When we have grace through the sacraments, we are better able to see our thoughts objectively because we have opened ourselves up to receive more of God's way of thinking.

For instance, the thought, "I'm too tired tonight, I'll skip Mass just one more time," may seem beneficial to you because your Passive Intellect thinks avoiding Church will buy you a well-deserved evening at home. But if you stop and reason with this thought through your Possible Intellect, you will realize that avoiding Church may provide temporary comfort, but will not result in your highest good. Of course it is easier to stay home. But this is the battle between good and evil. To do the hard thing, we must dwell in the Possible Intellect, to talk our will into doing what is right and virtuous.

It takes work to think about our thinking. This is why we journal, reflect, renounce, write down our food protocols, examine, and engage in the Great Experiment intentionally. It takes trial and error to get it right.

The goal of the mind is to know the Truth, and the goal of the will is to choose the good. This is why knowing the Truth, as informed by scripture and Tradition is so important for making sound moral decisions. When a moral thought and emotion are chosen by the will, then the Passive Intellect is updated, and this information is stored for the next time a similar situation comes around. This process forms neural pathways that result in virtues. When this is done over and over again, virtues are formed and vices are unwound.

In his book, *Our Thoughts Determine Our Lives*, Elder Thaddeus says, "All of creation—everything that exists on the earth and in the cosmos—is nothing but divine thought made material in time and space. Because we are made in the image of God, his energy and life is in us."

We are spiritual creatures. If we turn our thoughts and desires to communion with God and community with others, then we live our lives to the fullest. Attending daily Mass, weekly adoration, and monthly confession helps us to sort out our thoughts and receive grace to shift those thoughts toward love and abundance.

You may have gotten into the habit of watching Mass online, but it's time to get back into the physical Church building to partake of the sacraments and interact with people. What you will recieve from this effort will be nothing short of a miracle. Even the grand architecture within our Churches and Cathedrals will bless you. These are majestic examples of man's best effort to honor the life of Christ. In turn, Jesus uses the material things we encounter within the building to draw us to Him through our five senses. Music, incense, devout prayer, gestures, statues, altars, vestments, golden chalices, and so much more draw us into the Divine and pull us toward worship. It's no wonder God calls us back to the Church again and again.

Are you willing to commit to the sacraments and to regularly fellowship within the Church so that God can do the impossible with your life?

He's waiting for your "yes."

Go tell Him.

VIRTUOUS ACTIONS TO CREATE GOOD HABITS

In the space provided, reflect on the following questions:

How much time are you spending inside of the Church?

We know that thoughts are the root of all behavior. Be honest, what do you currently think about the Church?

What are some thoughts that would make you feel like coming to Church?

SPIRITUAL FASTING PRAYER: THE UNITY PRAYER

My adorable Jesus, May our feet journey together.
May our hands gather in unity. May our hearts beat in
unison. May our souls be in harmony. May our
thoughts be as one. May our ears listen to the silence together.
May our glances profoundly penetrate each other.
May our lips pray together to gain mercy from
the Eternal Father. Amen.

HOW OUR MIND WORKS

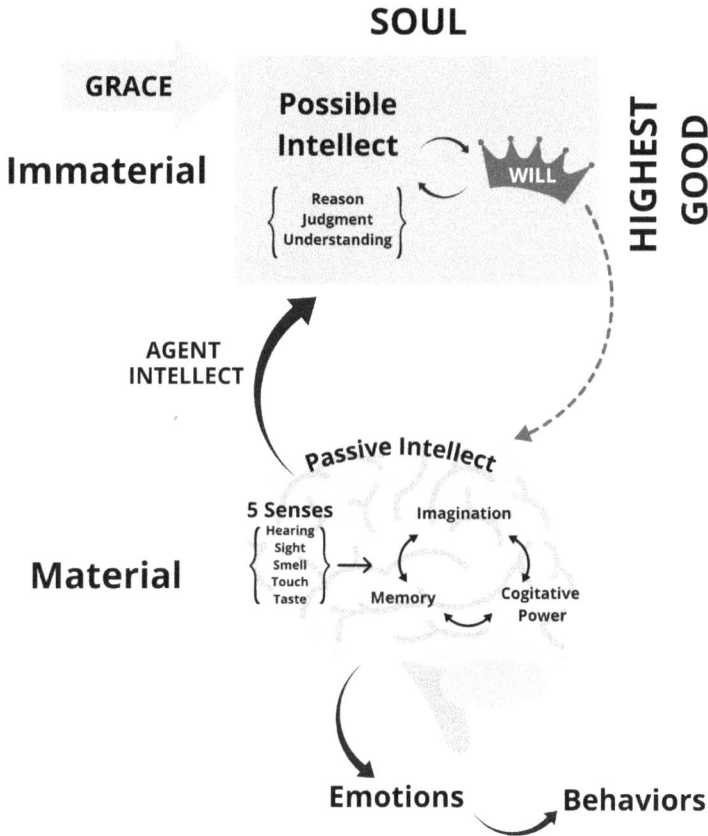

SOUL

GRACE

Immaterial

Possible
Intellect

Reason
Judgment
Understanding

WILL

HIGHEST
GOOD

AGENT
INTELLECT

Passive Intellect

5 Senses
Hearing
Sight
Smell
Touch
Taste

Imagination

Memory

Cogitative
Power

Material

Emotions   Behaviors

CONCLUSION

*"Be who God meant you to be
and you will set the world on fire."*

—St. Catherine of Siena[1]

God has a dream for you and me. But remember that everything worth doing is challenging at first. As you face the challenge of Spiritual Fasting, don't miss the sweetness along the way. Every Monday, when you plan your fasting, prayer, and almsgiving, you will be willingly led into the desert to forge a more simple life of contemplation. Then, as you meet the challenge and succeed in your intentions for the week, you will come out of that wilderness every Sunday with your heart and soul newly resurrected and ready to greet our Lord in a whole new way.

It's a reward much sweeter than sugar: a "little Easter" every week.

You see, Spiritual Fasting is never about what you give up. It's about what you gain as you become a person who can suffer well. As Pope Benedict XVI once said, "The world offers you comfort, but you were not made for comfort. You were made for greatness." If you want greatness, it's going to come with trials. It is the only way for God to show you what He will do for you if you believe.

One of my favorite stories in the Bible is found in Genesis 32, when Jacob wrestles God. I'd like to suggest that if you are not wrestling with God at this time, then your dreams are too small. Big dreams leave room for God. He loves working miracles that only He can take credit for, not you or me. Why? Because seeing the impossible drives more faith. And, faith gets us to heaven where we can be with Him eternally. Faith is not needed when life is easy. It only comes by struggle. But, be assured, the wrestling itself means that God is with you.

And He's not with you because you are doing things perfectly. I love how Chad Bird describes Jacob in his book, *Limping With God.*

> *"I thank God that he didn't choose a rule-following, t-crossing, i-dotting, cream of the moral crop, most-likely-never-to-do-anything-shameful man to be the patriarch of the OT people of God. He chose Jacob. He chose a disciple with a shady past, a troubling future, a dysfunctional family, and a heart drunk on ego to be his #1 guy. Christ wanted it to be patently clear that being his follower is not about climbing a ladder of spiritual success, but being greeted by Mercy at the bottom of the ladder by the Lord, who climbs down to us" (p. 69).*

Despite his questionable character, there was hope for Jacob, who was changed to Israel, meaning *one who contends with God.* Remember that your better self comes on the other side of the wrestling. If you are seeking a God of comfort then you will never change. He wants to contend with you. Spiritual Fasting is one way that He will do it.

The bottom line? Delay and Pray™ will change your identity.

That's what we need. Karol Wojtyla, before he was Pope John Paul II had this to say about the human person: "Man's interior life revolves around truth and goodness. The dynamism of desire is always open to redemption." In my life, the redemption of my desires looks like dreams that are coming to pass much differently than I expected. My dreams are so big that sometimes I think, "What am I doing?"

Lately, it all seems impossible.

I am wrestling God.

Every day, I am wrestling with Him by slowly but surely building a flourishing business out of nothing. I keep getting up before the sunrise and failing my way to success. I go to Mass daily, go to confession and adoration weekly, and pray. I tell God I am not leaving until He blesses me. And, He always does. Then I walk away to work another day. If I am limping as I go then He gets the glory. That's a good trade.

So I keep going when it's hard. I believe in His promise of Delay and Pray™ because I've seen it work. I just have to be patient as the good news of Spiritual Fasting reaches more people.

Fr. Jacob Meyer is an excellent example of the power of patience while wrestling for a dream. He is my nephew, and he has been a priest since 2012, but it would take ten more years before he reached a goal of being commissioned into the Navy as a chaplain. Getting fit had been a distant and impossible dream of his since he was young.

It was impossible because at the beginning of his priesthood, he reached his highest weight of 400 pounds. That made joining the Navy out of the question. Fr. Jacob knew his only hope was to surrender his desire to God.

He made some very tough decisions about his health, in both body and soul. He never gave up and failed his way to success one year at a time. God was with him as he wrestled. Eventually he used both medical means and Spiritual Fasting to lose the weight and enter into the Navy at a fit 200 pounds.

Fr. Jacob needed every experience that he went through to prepare him for what was ahead in the military. God knew the exact timing and the way it would happen. Fr. Jacob trusted Him, working hard, believing hard, praying hard, and waiting on the process. He had patience.

Before he left his parish, he was even given a key to the City of Mishawaka, Indiana by the mayor, declaring June 12th as Father Jacob Meyer Day. His example of faith was influential for his parish, the Diocese, and the city, as he served Catholics and non-Catholics alike.

What a beautiful ending to a chapter that Fr. Jacob thought would never change. Today, he would tell you that all of the waiting and wrestling was worth it.

Just like my nephew, the book of your life is not over. Spiritual Fasting will help you find and reach the dreams that God has written on your heart. Ask Him what they are. Form your new identity as you take care of your body as the holy temple that it is. This goes way beyond food.

It's as if we are saying, "Help me make space for You in the holy temple of my body. Come, Holy Spirit. Reside here. I want to be the Inn where the Holy Family can knock on the door of my heart and always be welcomed. I want to make space for truth and health and love."

The bigger your dreams, the more you prepare Him room.

COACHING TRANSCRIPTS

On the following pages, you will read several transcripts from Beth's coaching calls with her clients in the Delay and Pray™ Group Coaching Experience. These one-hour group calls are held online every week, where Beth teaches a mini-lesson and then opens the floor for anyone who would like additional help to understand themselves or get to the root of a thought that has been bothering them.

Access to coaching increases the success rate for Spiritual Fasters because they eliminate emotional distractions, enjoy the commitment and accountability that comes from community, and never have to go more than seven days without re-focusing on their optimal health goals.

These transcripts provide a broad sample of the types of questions and challenges that Spiritual Fasters encounter during the program.

COACHING TRANSCRIPT:
PRAYING FOR ADULT CHILDREN

Client: I hit a little bit of a struggle this week because I really miss my son.

Beth: *What's his story?*

Client: He's 28 and on his own. He has an almost four-year-old daughter. My problem is I don't get to see them because they say they're too busy. And so we had a little family meeting last month and talked about if and when we can have time with them, especially our grand-daughter. I just really miss him, and I have been praying for him like crazy. I am just sad, and therefore, I gave myself a free pass on my food this weekend. There is a lot of grief and sadness, and I am trying to turn it around and talk about it with the Lord, but ...

Beth: *So what does "a free pass on food this weekend" mean?*

Client: I ate quite a few carbs, and ...

Beth: *Can you quantify it?*

Client: Well, I ate some sourdough bread and some chips and treats. And some wine. I had three glasses, and I don't feel very good when I have that much. Oh, and I had some crackers ... and a piece of candy, last night.

Beth: *Okay. So what is the predominant thought about your son and the food, together?*

Client: I think it's kind of like, "why try?"

Beth: *"Why try" on the son or why try on the food?*

Client: I think both.

Beth: *"Why try" is a question. If you could put that question into a statement, what would that sound like?*

Client: It would sound like, "This hurts." It feels like a slap in the face from God about my son. A little backstory. He was very much a surprise pregnancy. I wasn't ready to be a mom so I never felt like I really bonded with him. So even though he has a great life, and we gave him a great childhood, I sort of think he may have felt rejection. I just felt really ill-equipped to be a mom, when he came into my world. I gave up a lot to have him. Pretty much my whole life … because I was on a trajectory. And just the way he treats me and us now is like, no gratitude, and I think, "Really God?"

Beth: *Yeah. So, obviously the feeling is sadness. Or is it anger? Which is heavier?*

Client: Sadness.

Beth: *So this weekend you were sad. And the action was you ate and drank more than you wanted to.*

Client: Yes, I just wanted to turn off the program for a while and deny that I am a part of Delay and Pray. I wanted to just be and eat.

Beth: *Is there any other action that came from sadness besides eating and drinking more than you wanted to and turning off the program?*

Client: No. I was responsible and went to church. I didn't crawl into bed and stay there. I engaged in life. But the part about food … that was the part that I just wanted to be and eat.

Beth: *So that tells us the food is the place where you are not showing up to feel your feeling of sadness. And that is common, right? Because it is hard to feel sad.*

Client: Well, and it's coupled with rejection, which is a deeper feeling. I know I made the right choice having him, but did I make the right choice raising him?

Beth: *You made the choice to raise him. He's 28 and has a four-year-old daughter. Would you say he has a pretty good life?*

Client: Yes, I do worry about his stress level. He owns his own company, and he says he is just too busy, and I get it. But I texted him twice this weekend, and I hadn't texted him in a month, and I left him a voicemail because his grandpa is not doing well, and there was no response. He didn't even acknowledge that I texted him or that he got a voicemail. That's all.

Beth: *That's good information to have. What percentage of your son can you control?*

Client: Zero … So I have to just accept this, and that's what I'm having a hard time doing.

Beth: *He came into this world as a surprise to you. And you did the most courageous and most unbelievable thing that you could ever do. You had him and you married his father and you raised him.*

Client: Thank you.

Beth: *What would it take, no matter what his response to you, to sit in absolute lovability for him?*

Client: It would take me getting past the grief of not spending time with him now and not making memories with my grand-daughter. That seems to be the block in the way.

Beth: *What if you can't see the future, and the future has that in it, but you just can't see it, yet?*

Client: Okay, that's what I feel the Lord is telling me, but it is hard to trust.

Beth: *What's interesting is that you're 100% lovable, no matter how your son treats you or responds. No matter what he gives you or how much time he spends with you. That's the first part. In the book Our Thoughts determine Our Lives, Father Thaddeus writes, "You don't have to love me; I love you all the more." What's beautiful about that is that it gives you tremendous peace. Then you can spiritually fast for your son and your granddaughter, and no matter what you are feeling, it is working. It's always working. Your intentions and spiritual fasting are always working. The Lord will give us consolations here and there, but even when we don't see them, it's always working. So you can reach into your heart and know that he loves you.*

Client: You mean, God, right?

Beth: *God and your son.*

Client: I have a hard time believing that my son loves me.

Beth: *What if you give him the benefit of the doubt that he does love you, he's just working through some things?*

Client: I guess I also have some fear. I have seen it happen to too many families that their children just cut them off. Especially with sons. They "leave and cleave" and don't even talk to the parents anymore. I'm kind of afraid that we are not going to make memories or be there on Mother's Day and birthdays. It will all just drift into Nowheresville, and I will be cut off. They have told me to stop sending gifts. I can't stop by. That was a disaster that happened last year. I've seen people cut other people out of their lives, and I have some fear of that.

Beth: *Then another thing we need to talk about is how useful is this type of fear that you are having?*

Client: None, I guess.

Beth: *Les Brown says "Fear is False Evidence Appearing Real." You know, you have never spiritually fasted like this before. What if this is new? What if you just leaned in with a little less anxiety and a little less worry, and you just started to sit at the feet of Jesus and know. To have a knowing that everything is going to be amazing in God's good time?*

Client: (laughs) I guess I would have to work on that.

Beth: *What if you do that and what if you forgive your son?*

Client: I don't have any ... something in particular?

Beth: *Yes, for not texting you back and not spending time with you.*

Client: Oh, I'm not mad at him. But I do think he may be getting a little pleasure out of punishing me.

Beth: *What if you stopped assigning motives to him and just went with the facts? He's 28. He owns his own business. He has a four-year-old daughter. What's the thought you want to think about him?*

Client: That God's got a plan for his life. I just want a friendship with him. I want to make memories. Go on walks or hikes. Have meals. Enjoy time together.

Beth: *Is that your spiritual fasting goal?*

Client: Yes.

Beth: *Until then, what are the thoughts you want to think of him?*

Client: Good thoughts. Happy thoughts. I know God has a plan for him.

Beth: *Do you think God has a plan for the two of you?*

Client: I hadn't thought of it that way.

Beth: *What about thinking God has a plan for both of you? I have a son, and I believe God has a plan for us. Try the thought, "God has a plan for us."*

Client: That's a little odd because we're a mother and son.

Beth: *No, it's not. I have a son, and I believe that God has a plan for us. He totally has a plan for us. My son and his wife live far away, and there are times when I feel sad. In the past I would eat or drink through the sadness, to take the edge off. But then I started praying, "Lord help me to feel this sadness." I would put my hand on my heart and say, "This is sadness. This is sadness." I just felt it. I would pray through the sadness instead of eating and drinking through the sadness. Eventually, sadness stopped bothering me so much. Now when my kids come for a visit and then leave, I notice sadness and think, "Oh this is sadness, and I want it." Why do I want sadness? Because I love my children so much, and it's an appropriate emotion to feel sadness when someone you love leaves. I love them so of course I am going to feel sad when they leave. I feel the sadness for a little bit, and then I pull up my bootstraps and get going the very next day. I do my best to love them from afar by sending them touch notes here and there. But my core belief is that God has a plan for each of my children, and I'm in it. No matter what is going to happen with my children in the future, I know that God will be with me providing and consoling, and I will never be alone. I even use my imagination to see us together here.*

Client: Hmmm ...

Beth: *I know that there will be reconciliation for you. You have to use your imagination to bring that into your thoughts. And also you have to forgive yourself. You have to forgive yourself for whatever you did or didn't do with your son. Sit in the glory of the fact that you gave birth to him. You made the decision to have him and raise him.*

Client: When my son was born, the doctor said, "This baby has an anointing on his life." And just last week I had a dream that he had a crucifix drawn on his back. I could see that he was marked by God. But he doesn't have faith anymore, and that is hard to watch. He is not even married. That feels like a rejection of everything I have taught him. It feels like a rejection of me.

Beth: *That's okay. Just say, "That's okay." The Lord is taking you through something that is going to glorify Him. You are going to show up a couple years down the road, telling a totally different story. But the Lord wants you to give it to Him first. So your son is rejecting you for now. He's finding himself. We've all been rejected by our kids at one time or another. I've been rejected by my own kids. All of them. We have to lean into the belief that they will come back. your son will come back one day. What's the downside of thinking that?*

Client: There isn't one.

Beth: *There isn't one. There is never a downside to thinking that God has a plan for us. In the meantime, your son doesn't have to love you. You can love him all the more.*

Client: I will.

COACHING TRANSCRIPT:
FEASTING ON SUNDAYS

Client: I have some drama for you. It's about Sundays.

Beth: *Let's hear it. What's happening with Sundays?*

Client: I do really great with all the rules for the week, and I know I can define what feasting on Sundays looks like. I think I don't want to define it so that I can continue to have permission to do whatever I want. Maybe I'm defining it by not defining it. I just want a healthy definition. I think it's weird not to be able to eat whatever I want on Sundays.

Beth: *But if you had to define it what would the definition be?*

Client: Probably eating whatever I want and giving in to every urge.

Beth: *So feasting equals eating whatever you want and giving in to every urge.*

Client: Yes.

Beth: *Your definition is just a thought. And if that is your thought then why are you surprised that you are eating whatever you want and giving in to every urge?*

Client: I'm not surprised at the result, but I don't want that result. But then I also don't want to discipline myself to have a different result. Does that make sense?

Beth: *Yes. You're saying you don't want to.*

Client: (laughs)

Beth: *So that thought—I don't want to—where is that coming from?*

Client: Well, the first thing that comes up in my mind is a sense of entitlement. Like, I've worked really hard all week, and I don't want to work hard anymore.

Beth: *Sundays are like your day off, your escape, your release.*

Client: Right. And I'm finding myself a little stressed right now because we are about to go on vacation, and I don't want to just open the gates to eat whatever I want.

Beth: *Of course you don't want to just open the gates.*

Client: But at the same time, I do.

Beth: *You have two competing thoughts right now. One is the thought: "I don't want to." And the other thought is: "I do want to." Of course the thought "I don't want to" is going to win out because that is the neural pathway that you already have in place. That's easy to see. It's the gluttony. It's the sloth. Even a Sunday is not a binge day.*

Client: I used to be much better at it. At first, it was easier. But now I find that I get to Saturday afternoon, and I am just done. I am all out of willpower. I don't write down what I am eating.

Beth: *So listen to your thoughts: I don't define feasting. I don't want to. I don't write down what I am eating.*

Client: I'm thinking those things because it's uncomfortable.

Beth: *Why is it uncomfortable?*

Client: Because my urges are stronger on the weekends, and it's harder to let those urges pass. I don't have as many urges during the week. That's just reality.

Beth: *Why do you think you have more urges on the weekend?*

Client: We are in celebratory mode on the weekends.

Beth: *You know your urges on the weekend are really about buffering. There is a feeling that you do not want to feel. You've just decided that you're not going to feel the feeling. That feeling doesn't have to be negative; it can be anything. It could be the feeling of celebration. You get to redefine celebration if you want to.*

Client: I'd like to, yeah.

Beth: *What would you like celebration to be?*

Client: It's helpful to make celebration mean connecting with other people.

Beth: *Okay, connecting with other people ...*

Client: Wait, so you're saying that I could be buffering with food to not feel a happy feeling?

Beth: *You are buffering with food to not feel a happy feeling. Think about it, when it is Friday night, you start wanting pizza or alcohol or* *desserts. That is what your brain thinks is celebration. For me, when I was just beginning to stop drinking on Friday nights, my brain would be screaming at me when I tried to drink only water instead. It would say, "This is not what we do! This is not what we do! We drink alcohol to celebrate on Friday nights!" That was the neural pathway I had created for years: Celebrate with alcohol and food. But you can diversify your celebration. I started walking around just saying to myself, "I delay sugar, flour, and alcohol to Sundays." Now my celebration is that I'm suffering for everyone on my prayer list. I'm delaying for everyone on my prayer list. I'm showing up in absolute joy. It's taken me a while to get here, but I use so many helpful things. I use music, I use podcasts, I use spiritual reading. I lean into the thought, "This is celebration. I'm celebrating that I can actually fast today."*

Client: I can understand that to some degree. But I still think that it's just wrong to delay or fast or limit myself on Sundays.

Beth: *If one of your children wanted to eat two hamburgers, three pieces of cake, four peanut butter cups, and a milkshake on Sunday, what would you say? And what if they begged you, arguing, "Mommy it's a Sunday! I'm supposed to be able to eat whatever I want on a Sunday!" Would you think it was a good idea for them?*

Client: Of course I wouldn't let them eat all of that on Sunday or any day.

Beth: *Of course you wouldn't. So my question to you is: What do you want to have on a Sunday? What would fuel you? What would be enough? What would be celebration in moderation?*

Client: Can you give me an example?

Beth: *Let's say I eat a cheeseburger, french fries and an ice cream cone. What's wrong with that?*

Client: Nothing.

Beth: *Nothing. Then tell me why I don't do it.*

Client: Maybe you don't need that anymore?

Beth: *Right, I don't need that anymore. It makes me feel sick. But that's not the main thing. The main thing is that now I don't want it. I don't want it anymore. I have told myself so many times that I am a person who can Spiritually Fast, and now it is easier than it used to be. But I cannot do it alone. I need the help of Jesus. So I am constantly asking Him, "Lord help me. Lord help me fast so I can pray for the people on my list. They need my prayers. They need my fasting. And I am willing to give it. I am constantly training my mind to want to. I am constantly training my mind to feast on other things. For instance we are going on vacation next week, and I have already planned out the way I will be feasting. I will be feasting on good books. I will be feasting on playing with the little kids in my extended family. I am even going to be feasting on my bathing suit. That may sound funny, but I bought a new bathing suit that is so adorable and fits me so well. I am going to enjoy that on my vacation. Sure, I have some special things planned to eat, and there is even alcohol on my plan. But food and drink are not the only ways I will be celebrating. Does that make sense?*

Client: It definitely makes sense. It just takes practice.

Beth: *Start writing it all down again so that you can look forward to it and enjoy it. You can plan it out, even on vacation. For instance, on my vacation I have already written down that every time we go out to eat I am going to choose a salad.*

Client: That makes me think of something worth celebrating! I may not be really excited about eating a salad, unless I focus on the fact that I didn't have to make it. Now, that feels like celebrating. I'm eating somebody else's grilled chicken salad that they made for me. That's a celebration right there.

Beth: *There you go!*

Client: When I say that, it feels like I'm allowing God's grace to touch all of it. Not just what's on the menu but every part of my life.

Beth: *That's right! We get to invite God's grace to touch all of it.*

Client: Yes.

COACHING TRANSCRIPT:
NOT HAVING ENOUGH TIME

Client: I am losing my resolve during the week, and I think it is because I am not writing down my protocol.

Beth: *Do you think or do you know?*

Client: Well, I know how effective protocol is but ...

Beth: *So why are you not doing it?*

Client: I don't think I have time. It's a little bit of a victim mentality that I am so busy right now. I have so many things going on, and I don't have enough time or bandwidth to add another "hard thing" to my pile. Even though I know the hard thing is going to yield benefits. That is one reason that I haven't raised my hand to get coaching in a while. I'm telling myself if I keep hiding then it will be okay. I can keep doing what I want to do.

Beth: *You're so normal. Just like all of us. The thought, "I don't have time" is interesting. Is it true, or is it a lie?*

Client: I think that thought a lot. Realistically, I guess it's a lie. I get the same amount of time as anybody else.

Beth: *So is it the truth, or is it a lie?*

Client: Well ...

Beth: *Is it the truth, or is it a lie?*

Client: It's a lie.

Beth: *The other day, I told my husband that the landscaper was going to charge $60. He actually charged $90. Later, I wanted to go back and tell my husband, "I didn't tell you the truth," but saying it that way is just a softened way of saying, "I told you a lie." I decided not to let myself off the hook so I said it like it was. I told my husband, "I told you a lie." That sounded shocking to him and to me, but he was able to forgive me right there on the spot. And I was able to forgive myself. He actually didn't care that it was $90. I don't know why I told him a lie. But then I started noticing all the times I am tempted to tell lies. And because I started noticing lies, I became hungry for truth. All I want is truth. I don't want to tell lies to others or to myself. What about you? Notice that you are telling yourself lies about your time. So, do you know why you are lying to yourself about time?*

Client: Why?

Beth: *Because you want to eat sweets.*

Client: (laughs) Yeah, I want to eat sweets!

Beth: *Why are you lying to yourself about the sweets?*

Client: Really? Okay, I want to eat these warm, fresh farmer's market cookies we've been picking up on Tuesdays. I do not want to delay them to Sunday. They are hot on Tuesday. But I could throw it in the freezer, I guess.

Beth: *How many souls could you save if you threw that cookie in the freezer? What if you were that powerful?*

Client: Well, I like power so I like the sound of that!

Beth: *We'll never know the value of that cookie until we get to heaven, will we? Can you imagine the power we are not utilizing? That's why sweets are so hard to give up. Because they have such consequence. Otherwise, it wouldn't be hard.*

Client: It's like I'm waiting for me to not want it. It's like I'm waiting for me to want to write everything down on my protocol.

Beth: *Although, another way to think of it is, "Thank God that I want this sweet. Because now I can offer it for all of the people I am praying for." I ask God to help me remember why I'm doing this. I don't wait for myself to stop wanting it. I ask for help to feel the discomfort instead of eating and drinking myself out of it. Don't forget the redemptive suffering.*

Client: Yep. That's the missing piece, right there. I have time. I am just afraid of the desire. I am afraid of the discomfort that the desire brings.

Beth: *Your soul can't afford for you to tell yourself the lie that you don't have time to write down your protocol.*

Client: Yes, I can tell that God is calling me to experience the desire, to embrace it, and not to satisfy it. Like you're saying, that's where the value is. To embrace the discomfort so that I can lean on Him through it. I'll do it. Thank you.

COACHING TRANSCRIPT:
STRUGGLING WITH CHANGE AND PERFECTION

Client: My daughter and her husband moved in with me temporarily. That is a challenge, and it is a transition. I know from past experience that I struggle with transitions. When there are too many changes around me, I feel like I can't meet my own expectations. So I'm trying to be gentle with myself in getting back to the Delay and Pray™ program. I haven't been following the program for the last month. Yesterday was the first day that I was able to go back on protocol.. But it's a miracle because I didn't gain any weight back, during that time, even with all my mess ups.

Beth: *Why do you think that is?*

Client: I think that I didn't gain weight this time because I lost the weight really slowly. The changes that I have made are changes that I can do.

Beth: *So tell me how your thoughts have shifted during this month of transition. What kinds of thoughts are you thinking?*

Client: Well, sometimes the negative thoughts come through, but I am able to recognize them and change them into more positive thoughts.

Beth: *Can you give me an example of a thought that comes up but now you are able to hold space for it and catch it. What thoughts are you taking captive with the Lord, asking His help to shift them?*

Client: It's mostly about perfection. For one thing, with two extra people in the house, the kitchen is messy. Thoughts about the messy kitchen are coming up. But you have taught me to leave room for things being different. So I have decided not to be upset when they leave their dishes in the sink or don't empty the dishwasher. I focus on things like, "I'm glad they are doing their own cooking and aren't expecting me to cook." I think to myself, "I have extra time in my schedule, and I can empty the dishwasher. It's not a big deal." So I am taking a more servant-hearted attitude toward it. I am not getting frustrated with the mess. It's different, and it's okay.

Beth: *I love it. So the thought is, "Things can be different, and that is okay." You know what's interesting? I can hear the calmness in your voice. There is a virtue at play here. Virtue is being infused in you that is enabling you to be servant-hearted. There is a virtue taking hold. What do you think that is?*

Client: Faith and perseverance. You know, a few days ago, I had an opportunity to support a ministry with a monthly donation, and I have never done this before, but I decided to do it. I have seen how powerful Spiritual Fasting is, and it made me want to increase my almsgiving. I thought, "Wow, what if I increase my almsgiving alone with the Spiritual Fasting, and then watch the Lord work." I was excited. It's opened up opportunities. This is opening me and everything around me. I am aware of the power of God and His angels.

Beth: *It truly is a three-fold cord: prayer, fasting, and almsgiving. When you actually commit to these things, the Lord is able to sow more virtue within your soul. You'll find the money to do all the things He's asking you to do. You'll find the time to do all the things He's asking you to do. You'll find the hunger to do all the things He's asking you to do.*

You'll find all the possibility in your life that He wants you to find so that you can pray, fast, and give.

Client: I did those things before but not so regularly. I'm seeing the power of consistency. There is still that sneaky tendency toward perfection. But I'm starting to believe that there is no "Throw-Away Day." Even if I mess up at the end of the day, all of the prayer and fasting that I did the first part of the day was not wasted. That's important for me to remember. Like, this Sunday, I feasted to "just enough" for breakfast and lunch. I was really proud of myself. But then at dinner, I had just been to a special Mass, and I felt lonely afterward. My daughter and her husband were not at home so I returned to an empty house. In that loneliness, I ate more than what was on my protocol. I wish I had been able to finish the whole day.

Beth: *Overeating is "under-feeling." You didn't want to feel that loneliness so you ate yourself out of it. Evenings can be a challenging time for a lot of us, as we are reviewing our experiences. One time, my husband said something unforgettable. He said, "Evenings are when I wander in the desert for 40 years … in the kitchen."*

Client: That's how I feel.

Beth: *So it would help to make a list of actions or behaviors that you could do in the evenings, but first you would need to make a list of thoughts you want to think in the evenings because we all know our actions originate in our thoughts. So what are the thoughts you want to think about walking into an empty house? Because that will happen again.*

Client: I could think, "I can spend my time however I want. I can choose what to do with my evening."

Beth: *How would you like to spend your evening? What would you like to do?*

Client: I could go for a walk. I could pray. I could sew or quilt. I could read.

Beth: *And what will you think when you fail at those planned behaviors? It's going to take a lot of "Nunc Coepis" in order for you to keep going and evolve into the plan that works for you.*

Client: It seems like it's all a matter of flexibility. I might have a plan, but if my daughter is sitting at the kitchen table and wants to talk, then I prefer to take that opportunity and postpone my plan.

Beth: *In fact, that action should be on your plan. Because your daughter is only with you for a short time. So enjoy the heck out of her.*

Client: Sometimes she stresses me out, though! But I noticed that thought the last time it came up. When I thought, "She's stressing me out!" I reasoned with myself, saying, "Well, if what she does can affect my level of stress, then maybe what I do can affect her level of peace."

Beth: *That's so true. But ultimately, she can't affect your level of stress. She doesn't have that power. You are letting her affect you. But that takes some practice. You are starting in the right place. Because you have decided that it's okay when things are different. It's okay when things change. It's okay when the kitchen is messier than usual. We can shift* *our thoughts by taking the crown of thorns and putting it around our own head for other people.*

Client: Yes. I can do that. Thank you so much.

ENDNOTES

Chapter 1: The Promise of Delay and Pray ™

1. Mark 12:31

2. Matthew 11:30

3. Lanteri, Venerable Bruno."Nunc Coepi". *Venerable Bruno Lanteri*, Accessed 5 Oct. 2023. https://www.omvusa.org/bruno-lanteri/about-bruno-lanteri/spirituality/nunc-coepi/.

4. Asher, Charles William and Dennis Patrick Slattery. *Simon's Crossing*. iUniverse, 2010.

5. Matthew 19:26

Chapter 2: Motivation for The Great Experiment

1. Chrysologus, Saint Peter. Sermon 43: PL 52, 320, 322.

2. Matthew 7:7

3. Weible, Wayne. *The Medjugorje Fasting Book*. Hiawassee, New Hope Press, 2009.

Chapter 3: Happy, Thin and Rich Right Now

1. "Novena to Blessed Pier Giorgio Frassati." *Catholic Doors Ministry*, https://www.catholicdoors.com/prayers/novenas/p03804.htm. Accessed 13 Dec. 2023.

2. Philippians 4:7

3. "Day 73. Sinners See With Eyes of Gratitude". *The 99 Day Novena*, Metanoia Catholic. https://www.99daynovena.org/novena/day-73. Accessed 13 Dec. 2023.

4. Most, Rev. William G."The Creation, Nature and Fall of Man". *EWTN Global Catholic Network*, Eternal Word Television Network Inc., 1990. https://www.ewtn.com/catholicism/teachings/creation-nature-and-fall-of-man-215. Accessed 18 Dec. 2023.

5. Catholic Church. *Catechism of the Catholic Church*. Catholic Cross Reference, 2024, https://www.catholiccrossreference.online/catechism/#!/search/2023-2024. Accessed 13 Dec. 2023.

6. 2 Corinthians 3:18

7. "Virtue of Mortification: Fr. Ripperger". YouTube, Sensus Fidelium, 31 July 2016. https://www.youtube.com/watch?v=6gsC9Kzuebk

8. Weible, Wayne. *The Medjugorje Fasting Book*. Hiawassee, New Hope Press, 2009.

Chapter 4: Believing Harder Than You Work

1. Roth, Geneen. *Women, Food, and God*. New York, Simon and Schuster, 2010.

2. Isaiah 55:8-9

3. Matthew 19:26

4. Barbaric, Fr. Slavko. *Pray With The Heart!* Information Center MIR Medugorje, 2003.

Chapter 5: The Thought Model of Possibility with God

1. *Pastoral Constitution on the Church in the Modern World Gaudium Et Spes Promulgated by His Holiness*, Pope Paul VI, Section 24, 7 December 1965.

1. Paul IV. Gaudium et Spes. December 7, 1965. Papal Archive. The Holy See. https://www.vatican.va/archive/hist_councils/ii_vatican_council/documents/vat-ii_const_19651207_gaudium-et-spes_en.html (paragraph 24).

2. Traherne, Thomas. *Centuries of Meditations*. Christian Classics Ethereal Library. 1908. https://www.ccel.org/t/traherne/centuries/cache/centuries.pdf

Chapter 6: Dining in with Jesus

1. Stephens, Gin. *Fast. Feast. Repeat.* St. Martin's Griffin, 2020.

   Hamilton, Jon. "Think You're Multitasking? Think Again." *National Public Radio*, 2 Oct. 2008, www.npr.org/templates/story/story.php?storyId=95256794.

2. Philippians 4:7

Chapter 7: Lots of Sugar and a Little Fiber

1. Tiwari;, Aditi, and Palanikumar Balasundaram. "Public Health Considerations Regarding Obesity—Statpearls—NCBI ..." *National Library of Medicine*, 5 June 2023, www.ncbi.nlm.nih.gov/books/NBK572122/.

2. "Adult Obesity Facts." *Centers for Disease Control and Prevention*, Centers for Disease Control and Prevention, 17 May 2022, www.cdc.gov/obesity/data/adult.html.

3. Jeff Krasno, "Mindful Eating to Digest Better, Feel Great, & Lose Weight". One Comune, Episode 313, July 21, 2022. https://www.onecommune.com/blog/podcast-mindful-eating-to-digest-better-feel-great-lose-weight-with-dr-siva-mohan-dr-mary-pardee-dr-jim-gordon-dr-pedram-shojai-kimberly-snyder-and-jason-wrobel

4. Lustig, Dr. Robert. *Fat Chance*. Plume, Penguin Group, 2014.

5. Steen, Juliette. "Exactly Why Sugar and Fiber Intake Is the Key to Weight Loss." *HuffPost*, HuffPost, 21 Apr. 2017, www.huffpost.com/entry/so-this-is-exactly-how-sugar-makes-us-fat_n_61087603e4b0999d2084f42d#:~:text=Because%20what%20we%20eat%20(sugar,to%20it%2C%22%20Lustig%20explained.

"Does Body Weight Affect Cancer Risk?" *American Cancer Society*, 15 Dec. 2023, www.cancer.org/cancer/risk-prevention/diet-physical-activity/body-weight-and-cancer-risk/health-issues.html.

"What Is the Gut? It's Time To Meet Your Gut." *The Gut Stuff*, 8 Apr. 2022, thegutstuff.com/intro-to-the-gut/get-to-know-the-gut/.

6. Barbaric, Fr. Slavko. *Pray With The Heart!* Information Center MIR Medugorje, 2003.

Chapter 8: Feasting on Life

1. Richards, Jay W. *Eat, Fast, Feast: Heal Your Body While Feeding Your Soul-a Christian Guide to Fasting: How Science Is Validating an Ancient Practice*. HarperOne, 2020.

2. Bernard, Saint. "Saint Bernard Quotes." *Brainy Quotes*, www. brainyquote.com/quotes/saint_bernard_778622. Accessed 28 Dec. 2023.

Emmons, D.D. "Understanding the Church Calendar: Simply Catholic." *Simply Catholic*, Our Sunday Visitor, 21 July 2023, www.simplycatholic.com/understanding-the-church-calendar/. Accessed 28 Dec. 2023.

"Solemnities, Feasts and Memorials." *Our Lady of Hope Parish*, The Catholic Community of Grafton, MA, ourladyofhopegrafton. org/solemnities-and-feasts. Accessed 28 Dec. 2023.

3. John 14:6

4. "A Prayer Before Fasting." *The Catholic Crusade*, www. thecatholiccrusade.com/a-prayer-before-fasting.html. Accessed 18 Dec. 2023.

Chapter 9: The Vice and Virtue Cycles

1. Lembke, Dr. Anna, MD. *Dopamine Nation*. Dutton, 2021.

2. "Bishop Baron on Knocking Holes in the Buffered Self: Approaches to the Question of God". YouTube, uploaded by Bishop Robert Barron, 30 Oct. 2020, https://www.youtube. com/watch?v=QvvDcII_2bM.

Chapter 10: The Answer is in the Church

1. Chrysologus, St. Peter, "Prayer Knocks, Fasting Obtains, Mercy Receives". St. John the Evangelist Catholic Church, Sermon 43: PL 52, 320, 322, Waynesville, North Carolina, 2018.

2. Fournier, Deacon Keith. "Good Friday, the Passion and the

Church." *Common Good*, 15 Apr. 2017, commongoodonline. org/good-friday-the-passion-and-the-church/.

"Importance of Management: Question." *Toppr*, Haygot Technologies, 2003, www.toppr.com/ask/question/the-definition-that-has-been-criticized-as-gospel-of-mammon-a-pig-science-etc-is/.

Catholic Church. *Catechism of the Catholic Church*. Catholic Cross Reference, 2024, https://www.catholiccrossreference. online/catechism/#!/search/2023-2024. Accessed 13 Dec. 2023.

Smiljanic, Ana, and Elder Thaddeus of Vitovnica. *Our Thoughts Determine Our Lives: The Life and Teachings of Elder Thaddeus of Vitovnica*. St. Herman of Alaska Brotherhood, 2010.

Schuchts, Bob. Be Transformed: *The Healing Power of the Sacraments* . Ave Maria Press , 2017.

Conclusion

1. St Catherine of Siena. *"Quotable Quote."* Goodreads, www. goodreads.com/quotes/20893-be-who-god-meant-you-to-be-and-you-will. Accessed 29 Dec. 2023.

2. Bird, Chad. *Limping with God: Jacob & the Old Testament Guide to Messy Discipleship*, 1517 Publishing. Irvine, CA, 2022, p. 69.

ACKNOWLEDGMENTS

This book is only being published because of the amazing people who made it happen when I first learned of life coaching, and I want you to know them!

The first person I must thank is Brooke Castillo from The Life Coach School. I discovered her podcast way back in 2016, and my life was forever changed by her beautiful energy and love for mindset work and by learning and applying the concept of the Thought Model to food consumption. It was at LCS that I met fellow coach and writer extraordinaire, Nika Maples. She is my ever-smiling and bubbly publishing team! My Jesus-loving friend and book coach rolled all into one. I thank her from the bottom of my heart for sticking with me for almost two years to get this book written and published! It is a gem.

It wasn't enough just to learn the Thought Model, I had to find the Catholic basis behind it. Many thanks go out to Matt and Erin Ingold, the husband and wife team/founders of Metanoia Catholic. Both deeply spiritual and humorous, they certified me as a Catholic Coach, and taught me all I know about the body-soul composite, deepening all I learned about the Thought Model into the Reason Cycle. They are why I am first a Catholic Mindset Coach turned Spiritual Fasting Coach! I feel such love and gratitude for all the people and coaches from both The Life Coach School and Metanoia Catholic—I can live out my mission because of all of you!

Special shout out to those of you who worked so hard with me to get my business started, out of which this book is a product: Kara at Plan-it Earth Marketing, Brittany at That Creative Girl, Lisa

Canning, Michelle Dunne, Shane Frost at Momentum Marketing, Dr. Amruti Choudhry, Albert Saenz, and Teresa Eppich. Where would I be without your initial support!

A huge thanks goes out to Jay W. Richards, author of *Eat, Fast, Feast: Heal Your Body While Feeding Your Soul*. He gave me the idea of using a regimen as a Rule of Life to make Spiritual Fasting much easier to wrap your mind around. He's brilliant and funny—a great person and resource for everything fasting!

Most importantly, I'd like to thank my amazing team at The Catholic Fasting Coach for all they do every single day of the year to keep me running: Kristina, Dani, and Joann. I couldn't have a business without your skills, talents, and friendship. Also, my star clients who constantly lend their voices and testimonials of their amazing progress through the program and in this book: Nikki, Jackie, Jenay, and Stefanie. Your determination and willingness to fail in order to get to success is inspiring.

Deepest gratitude goes out to my husband and children—my wonderful family who consistently offer all their love and support in my pursuit of this crazy Life Coaching journey (including this book) as well as seeing me through the ups and downs of learning how to spiritually fast and build a business on my own. The love, creativity, business knowledge, and graphic design skills of this family have helped me so much. I love you all!

I thank my sisters, Julie and Carolyn, who were my first students, my guinea pigs, best supporters, and my first testimonials! You are both sisters and friends, keeping me humble and laughing at all times. I love you so much. I also thank all my other siblings and parents (on both sides of the family) for giving me the best family ever to grow up in.

I thank God and the Blessed Mother for my Catholic faith, for which I am indebted.

I thank Father Jacob Meyer, who leads by example, is bold and courageous, and has always encouraged me to pursue this Spiritual Fasting dream. I thank the countless other priests and friends from my parishes who have influenced and encouraged me along the way as well.

And finally, a huge, thank you to all of my clients, who have hired me to coach them, trusted me to lead them, and are brave enough to stay in the battle of Spiritual Fasting. Some of the fruits of your efforts are visible here on earth, but the big stuff will be revealed to you in heaven! Keep going!

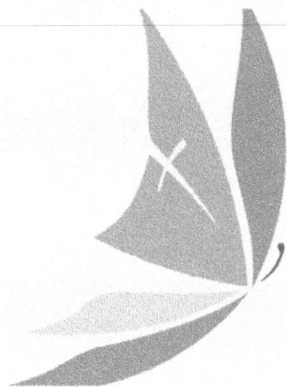

STOP. LET'S TAKE A
breath.

You are being invited onto a new and wonderful weight loss path.

This journey of health will actually get you where you want to go because you will be **holding the hand of Jesus** while learning to delay unhealthy foods and pray for others through it all.

You will drop the weight for good and find **joy in the challenge**, too.

....

Visit us at
www.thecatholicfastingcoach.com to learn how you can start your journey to a healthier and holier life.

Scan this code for a **FREE** 7 Day Meal Plan to jumpstart your spiritual fasting!

GET TO KNOW

Beth

·········· ·········

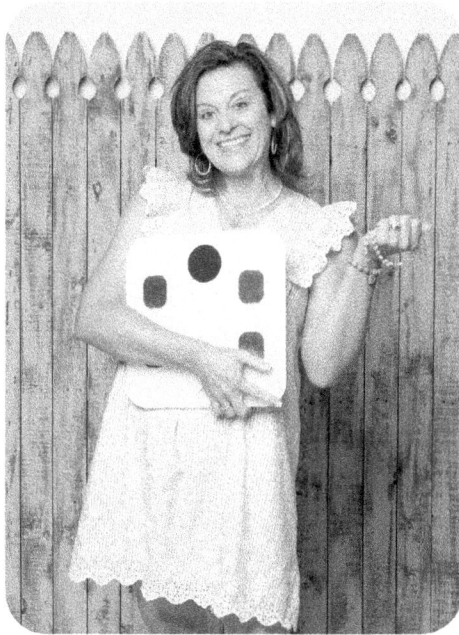

www.thecatholicfastingcoach.com

··················

f @thecatholicfastingcoach ⬡ @thecatholicfastingcoach

The Spiritual Fasting Guide with 7 Day Meal Plan

Scan this code for a **FREE** 7 Day Meal Plan to jumpstart your spiritual fasting!

https://catholicfasting.kartra.com/page/bookresource

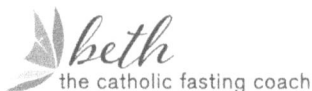

beth
the catholic fasting coach

www.ingramcontent.com/pod-product-compliance
Lightning Source LLC
Chambersburg PA
CBHW052019030426
42335CB00026B/3199